The Psychology of Cyber Dating

Discover the Secrets to Successful
Internet Dating and Learn to Improve
Your Love Life, Your Sex Life, and
Intimacy in Your Relationships

ROBERT DAVENPORT

authorHOUSE®

AuthorHouse™
1663 Liberty Drive
Bloomington, IN 47403
www.authorhouse.com
Phone: 1-800-839-8640

First published by AuthorHouse 6/22/2010

ISBN: 978-1-4520-1522-4 (sc)

Printed in the United States of America
Bloomington, Indiana

This book is printed on acid-free paper.

Cover design by Paul Harman,
moonship27@yahoo.com

Dedication

This book is dedicated to my beautiful and loving wife Rose who without her, this book would not even be possible, and our precious gift from GOD...our daughter Faith who we both love, adore, and treasure so dearly, we are so blessed to have her in our life...Thank You God! And our other four legged kids; Cindy aka "Grandma" our beautiful blonde Shar-pei / Yellow Blonde Lab who Rose and I rescued in Fall of 2000 from an animal shelter and is famous for her big smile and purple tongue hanging out the side of her mouth, next we have Mr. Mooshie who is our beloved "fatty-boom-boom" king of the house cat, then we have Sweetie who is our lovely Blonde Pomeranian mixed with White Poodle (who together with Cindy we nick-named Blonde and Blonder) and last but certainly not least we have Brody who is the newest terrorist in the house. Brody is what we call a "Poma-Cher-Ranian" (which is a mix of Pomeranian, Chiwawa, and Jack Russell Terrier) and is an absolute terrorist to the others. I dedicate this book to them for all the hours they had to sacrifice not having my attention to help them and look after them. It is because of your sacrifices that this book could manifest into reality. I love each of you so very much and every one of you have brought a special gift in to my life with your presence. Thank you!

Contents

Foreword

As we gaze up into the stars, and look past our distant planets and galaxies, and way beyond the new star formations, and even past the heavens, and as far as time can see, we eventually come to the stark realization, that when it is all said and done, we have to accept the fact that even though we are surrounded by billions of other people on planet earth, we are ultimately here alone all by ourselves. For most people this is a very disturbing and uncomfortable truth.

To embrace this truth and know that at some point throughout our lives, each of us will have to accept and come to our own realization that ultimately we are here all alone and by our self, that is a GIVEN, BUT that by accepting and allowing the realization of being alone to become our ultimate destination, is our CHOICE! The answer to this challenge of being alone is in the discovering and realization that we do ultimately have a CHOICE about everything including whether or not we end up being alone and by ourselves or discovering and walking down our life's path creating, having, and enjoying ideal relationships in our life.

It is my desire to share with you some of my own personal experiences throughout this book. In detailing some of the very choices and life lessons that I had to experience and learn along the way I will explain to you exactly what I did so that I would ultimately end up having the ideal relationship of my dreams. Through these experiences and lessons that I am now willing to bring public and share with you, I have been able to discover the most wonderful person halfway around the globe, and as a result, I now have my ultimate dream relationship with my loving and beautiful wife, Rose.

I hope that the lessons and real life examples contained in this book can help as many people around the world as possible learn to have a greater sense of understanding of how ANYONE that really wants to, can CHOOSE to have the ideal relationships that they so desire and crave for and that this book will help lead them to that wonderful and exciting discovery.

For the purpose of getting the absolute most out of this book, it is best if you view the content in this book as a portal or gateway of knowledge and information that you can continually come back to and review as often as you need to. Viewing the book this way will help the reader learn how to better transcend their understanding of the importance of CHOICES in relationships for the better, AND will teach you how to safely and successfully include the internet as a way to help expand your choices for meeting the right types of people that you want to have in your life.

So remember to pick up this book often and continue to read it throughout your life so that you too may learn and be prepared to successfully meet, greet, and embrace those wonderful undiscovered relationships and in the process end up having the fun and loving relationships that you so desire and crave for deep down inside.

Welcome to..."The Psychology Of Cyber Dating".

Introduction

Congratulations on making a great decision to invest in yourself and to begin improving on all of your relationships by purchasing and reading this book. Everyone will have their own individual personal reasons for wanting to pick up and read this book. For example: Have you ever been on a date and not known what to say or do next, or did not know how to take your new relationship to the next level? Or wasn't even sure how to go about getting a date? If so, then this book was designed for you and will share with you many important facts and ideas on how to strengthen and further all of your relationships from now on. Perhaps your reason for wanting to read this book is because maybe you are looking for the right words to say or how express yourself or maybe the right way to say the words, or maybe you just want your relationships to be more meaningful, or perhaps you just simply want to avoid the possibility of being embarrassed on your next date.

Either way, this book will open up new directions and possibilities that you can start using immediately to take your relationships in a newer and more exciting direction. You ultimately do have AND always will have a CHOICE. Above all else, for your own safety and success, remember this one very important fact: YOU HAVE A CHOICE! Do not feel pressured in to doing ANYTHING you are not comfortable with or certain about. Too many people have already ended up dead or missing because of failure to keep safety as their number one concern. Safety should always be your number one concern when you meet, greet and embrace people through the internet, regardless of what you want the outcome to be. So if you are ready to begin your new and exciting journey learning to have or keep the ideal relationship(s) of your dreams...let's begin!

I personally met my wife through the Internet on July 15th 2000 and we will be celebrating our 10th Anniversary on September 16th 2010. Coming from first-hand experience in meeting, greeting, embracing, dating, and finally marrying my ultimate marriage partner, I felt it would be best to have this type of book written by someone such as myself who has actually experienced life's ups and downs of marriage and divorce and meeting, greeting and dating people through the Internet, and be able to present these experiences to you in real life terms that are easy to understand, apply, and follow.

With all of these ups and downs and disappointments and knowledge gained from all of my experiences, I felt that it would also be helpful to include some psychological factors in this book that will help you understand and learn the best and most successful ways for meeting, greeting, and embracing people through the Internet. This information applies to anyone interested in using the Internet to help them look for their very first date, an ideal marriage partner, or someone to just be friends with, and will also cover the best ways to maintain all of your existing relationships in the process.

While you are reading and learning, I am going to be sharing some important and valuable information that will be helpful for you each step of the way. I will do this by making some suggestions, and coaching you on what to do when you find yourself in certain social situations. I will also be sharing some of my own actual experiences which you can begin using for discovering and improving your ideal relationships starting the same day your read it. You will find this information easy to understand, apply and follow in your day-to-day life.

Whatever your personal reasons are for wanting to read this book, please relax and enjoy reading because you are about to learn the best there is to know about "The Psychology Of Cyber Dating". So whether you are looking for a friend, a dating partner, a lover, a soul mate or an ideal marriage partner, this book will cover both how to use the internet and some of the psychology behind human actions, emotions, and behaviors which will help you find and keep the right relationship(s) in your life. I will also be sharing some information on seven different people that I personally met through the Internet. This includes relationships ranging from friendship to casual sex, to long-term dating and eventually to marriage.

Did you realize that with everybody having such a busy schedule and now having mobile internet access, using the Internet can be one of the best and safest ways of finding and meeting people without putting yourself at risk or totally embarrassing yourself in public? Best of all, you will not have to go and spend a fortune hanging out a bars and clubs hoping to accidentally bump into the "right person" or have to deal with obnoxious and drunk people falling all over you. This book focuses in on helping you successfully find the right type of person for yourself. You will also learn what you should look for in an online profile, the best approach to use when initiating contact with someone of interest for the very first time, what to say the first time you initiate contact, how to transition from initial contact to meeting in person, when and where are the best times and places to meet and most importantly ways to help protect yourself at all times.

Please bare in mind that meeting new people over the internet is still very risky and should be approached with extreme caution. I honestly believe that most of the people posting classified ads over the Internet are sincere and have good intentions. Some however, are out to play games and take advantage of other people. By reading this book and having a better understanding of how to identify and meet the right types of people through the Internet, you will be better equipped to set your goals and quickly proceed with confidence in meeting the right person or persons. Again, please understand that reading this book is no guarantee and that you are in fact taking a risk by deciding to meet someone over the internet, and that each decision you make and each step you take must be done with extreme caution.

Now, some of the benefits that you will learn and gain from reading this book include:

1. More effective ways to meet people through the Internet
2. Where some of the best places are to meet new friends through the Internet
3. What to look for in someone's online profile
4. Ways to better understand someone's online profile
5. Ways to verify someone's online profile

6. How to begin an effective dialogue with someone of interest

7. Ways to minimize your risk of being taken advantage of

8. When are the best times to transition from chatting to meeting in person

9. What are the best ways to have someone agree to initially meet you in person

10. Where are some of the best places to initially meet in person for romantic relationships

11. What you can do to best protect yourself when you do meet with someone for the very first time in person

12. How to establish rules for meeting someone in person and knowing when to say "Times Up"

13. When to decide if it is time to move on and not get involved without hurting someone's feelings...and last but certainly not least.

14. Understanding the psychology behind relationships and how to use this new knowledge to improve your existing relationships and create better and longer-lasting new ones.

Please understand that for the purposes of this book, the word relationship will be used a lot and applies equally to friendships as well as romantic relationships depending on what your goals are.

If you notice that you are having any difficulty or problems in any of your relationships, please feel free to refer back to this book and read up on the important lessons contained within the psychology section. You really can have the ideal relationship(s) or find the dream person that you have always been searching for. The key is to completely understand the right way to go about meeting them, and then understanding the secret of knowing how to keep them. That is exactly what the lessons in this book will help teach you.

While this book can be used to help you discover new relationships, it can also be used to help improve existing relationships that you might already be involved in and are not ready to give up on. Please share this book with your partners involved in your relationship(s) and let them know how much you love and care for them and that you would like for the two of you to read this book so that you can work on improving and strengthening your relationship together.

Chances are, one of the following lessons should help correct any problems that you are experiencing in your relationships. My personal wish for you is that this book will help you uncover and learn the missing pieces in your relationships and in return allow you to better understand and function in all of your relationships more successfully. Please keep in mind that this is the very first book I have ever written and that I fully expect there may be some grammatical errors and misspelled words. Please be understanding and forgive me of any of these mistakes that you may find as you read on and if you would be kind enough to please bring any mistakes to my attention by emailing them to psychologyofcyberdating@gmail.com or contact me through the website at www.PsychologyOfCyberDating.com Thank you!

Chapter 1:

"My Personal Experiences"
"Learning from my mistakes"

In January of 1998, my ex-wife and I really began to have some major personal marital problems before we filed for divorce. There were a number of factors and people that contributed to our problems but the main reason is because I was extremely busy working on several business ventures and partying with my friends more than I should have and the two combined together consumed about 90% of all my time, which ultimately left her feeling lonely and I can only imagine unappreciated most of the time. Looking back I realize where I made a lot of the wrong CHOICES.

The ironic part about my situation is that I was working very hard and was spending so much time towards achieving something so great in an effort to be able to shower my ex-wife in gifts, a beautiful home, and fine dining that my lack of time spent with her ended up being the reason for us splitting apart. Let me repeat this...the fact that we had very little time together ended up being one of the main reasons we started and ended up splitting apart.

I wanted to be able to give my wife everything she could have possibly ever wanted and was determined to work day and night until I achieved it, only to realize that she was not going to be around to enjoy those fruits of such long and intense labor. Being Asian and very set in her ways, she had decided that 3 ½ years of marriage with me in this situation was enough and that she wanted to move out and move on with her life.

1

Needless to say, I was devastated! In a FLASH, our lives together, my drive, my passion, our plans were suddenly flipped upside down and I felt like I was in a slow motion free-fall and the pain in my heart just lingered on and on and there was nothing I could do to stop it. When the dust settled and I finally was able to catch my breath, it was too late! Just like a vacuum being turned on, everything I was working for and looking forward to was completely sucked out of my life in what seemed like an instant!

I guess I was raised the old fashioned way because I was taught to believe that when you marry someone, you marry them for better or for worse and that you stick by each other's side and work things out no matter how difficult the problems may appear, you're together for life. According to the way my parents raised me, divorce was not an option. Certainly, I was committed to staying together and resolving our problems, but apparently, my ex-wife decided that she had had enough, and just like that, we were divorced. No amount of pleading or crying or explaining was going to change her mind. She was set in her ways. The real sad part was that I made assumptions and took things for granted with regard to our communication. Looking back, I now realize that with the two of us learning to be a little more effective in our communication, we very likely could have worked things out between us.

As it turns out, she had met someone through the Internet while we were still together. One Saturday afternoon in April of 1998, she decided to take off driving to go see this new person she met through the Internet who was located in another State. After having an extra-marital affair with this person, she returned home 2 days later. Confessing to me what she did, and we both decided that it was pretty much over between us.

To add even more sting to the punch I just received, she had set in her mind that she was going back to this person that she had met over the Internet and had committed adultery with, to live with him and start a new life with him and his 3 kids. As it turns out, he had just lost his wife the same exact way...cheating on him with someone she had met over the Internet. He must have did a reality check because he told my ex-wife that he did not want to be with her because he still needed time to get over the recent loss of his own wife cheating on him and leaving him. Needless to say by this point, my ex-wife was really devastated by his news and was not able to continue in her new relationship with him as a result. Isn't it funny how things turn out? Karma was coming full circle very quickly this time.

So imagine for a minute now...here is this scumbag portraying himself through the Internet as being somebody nice, romantic, sincere, and kind-hearted who is preying on innocent victims browsing the Internet and as it turns out, he's actually a single father of 3 small children living in a poor run-down town and barely able to keep his electric turned on, and put food on the table, and whose wife has just dumped him for somebody she met on the Internet. This is only a small snapshot of the types of people that are on the Internet that you must be aware of and protect yourself against.

Please understand, he never had any intentions of loving or caring for my ex-wife. All he wanted was to prove to himself that he could convince someone innocent and weak to fall into his trap. My ex-wife, being at a point of vulnerability and impressed with his online profile, fell into his trap and in the end became his victim. Communication, which is one of the main topics covered in this book, could have prevented this pain and the devastation through proper marriage counseling.

By the first part of June, 1998, my ex-wife and I had signed our final separation papers. She moved out of my house and moved in with some friends of mine until it was time for her to fly out across the United States to meet up with someone else that she had met over the Internet. That decision did not turn out too well for her either. Apparently, she did not understand the art of meeting people through the Internet, nor how to protect herself in the process.

You can only imagine that this was one of the most difficult and trying times of my entire life. I loved this person so much and would have done practically anything in this world for her. In my eyes she was the sunshine of the day, the beautiful scenery, and all of the wonderful sounds in life wrapped up in one, and in my eyes she could have done no wrong. She was such a gentle and loving and caring person...and suddenly, just like that, she had been taken away from me.

I felt as though my breath had been literally taken away from me and no matter how much or how deep I breathed, I still felt like I was suffocating. I remember so many nights being home alone laying on my bed crying and reflecting through everything that had happened in our relationship. The good times and the bad, I remember suddenly feeling confused and asking myself...what is this life all about? Why me? Where did I go wrong? What could I have done differently that would have made things better? Will she ever come back to me? All I really ever wanted was a simple, down-to-earth life with my wonderful wife.

To this day, I still sit and sometimes reflect back on some of the times that we spent together while we were still married and how truly wonderful and beautiful those precious moments really were. Treasure those moments and time you get to spend together, because just like with me, they can be gone in a FLASH. I can still see her standing in front of the mirror putting on her makeup or chasing after me to tickle me, and seeing her observing a beautiful butterfly as if it were a brand new miracle that she had never seen before. I often think to myself...I would give anything in this world to be able to go back in time and change the bad moments and do things differently. I should have CHOSE to do things differently. From this great lesson, I have learned to realize that ultimately it is MY CHOICES that will determine my outcome. That only I can be held accountable for my decisions and actions which led me to where I was at that point in my life, and that I could only blame myself and accept full responsibility for what happened and what will continue to happen throughout my life. Likewise, the same is true for YOU!

I know that I will never have the opportunity to make good on what happened in our relationship. Even though at the time, I had the best of intentions while we were together, I failed to properly communicate these intentions to her so that she would feel like she was a part of what I was doing and vice versa. So if you gain nothing else out of reading this book, please learn from some of my obvious mistakes, be proactive and learn to effectively communicate with each other.

I know that we all sit back from time to time and wonder about our purpose in life and our reason for being here on Earth and the many challenges we must face and go through every single day. It is only natural for us to wonder about these things. To this day, I still miss her and will always have love for her in my heart no matter how she feels towards me. I simply do not know how to just suddenly stop loving someone that I cared for so much.

She could look me straight in the eyes and tell me how much she hated me and I would still love her. But that is long gone and in my past and now I have a wonderful and beautiful wife, an incredible daughter, four of the most precious pets you can image and a beautiful home! Everyday I wake up I feel on top of the world and sometimes have to pinch myself to remind myself that it is real. Because of my own CHOICES and focus, I have the most incredible life that anyone could ever wish for, and it was created all by design, all because of my CHOICES.

As far as I know, to this day my ex-wife is still struggling with her decisions in life both financially and emotionally and probably still has not found her Mr. Perfect and unless she learns these lessons, probably never will. I often wondered if she had lost touch with reality from watching so many Soap Operas on TV and thinking that there really was such a life to live as those portrayed on the Soaps. I truly wish her good Luck in finding that special someone in her life that she deserves.

Since filing for our separation and waiting for the divorce to finalize, I took some well-needed time off from being in relationships to evaluate my values, morals and thoughts. It's amazing what you can discover and learn when you are finally ready to learn. You know how the old saying goes..."The teacher will appear when the student is ready." Well you can only imagine how ready I was to learn and pick up the broken pieces of my life and move forward as fast as I can.

Amazingly, after months of feeling lonely, confused, frustrated, and full of anger over this emotional tornado that just ripped apart my life and my dreams, I remember walking into my home-based office and finding a book sitting on my bookshelf that for some strange reason caught my attention. The amazing part is that after picking up the book and flipping through it, I could not recall ever purchasing this book, nor how it got on my bookshelf. The title was very intriguing and so I immediately began reading the first chapter and was completely overwhelmed with what I was learning from this new book.

It was as if this book was somehow mysteriously placed on my bookshelf and was written specifically for me to teach me how to deal with my anger and emotions that were bottled up inside of me from what I had just experienced in my marriage and divorce with my ex-wife. The more I read, the more intrigued I became. Every chapter dealt with some facet of my life that I seemed to be struggling with. It seemed as if God had intervened somehow by putting this book in front of me that showed me how to deal with and begin improving on my situation.

Needless to say, finding this book was a very welcome surprise for me, and the turning point for this enormous amount of grief and anger I had built-up inside. Suddenly for the first time in almost six months, I could laugh and feel joy inside again. I was no longer mad at the world and was beginning to see life in a new and improved way. Going through this type of experience has an unforgiving way of making me humble. I developed the ability to begin paying attention to the smaller things in life that are important while being able to overlook and just smile at the less important larger things.

I found myself being not so concerned anymore with who was right or wrong about a certain topic or subject because that was not what was really important, rather I now found myself happy just being there surrounded by loving and caring people. I learned not to be so pushy, rather except things the way they are at that moment and realize that through your intentions and desires coupled with faith and belief in yourself, you could eventually change the outcome through your intentions and actions. I learned that embracing uncertainty in our everyday life is extremely healthy and satisfying to our spirit. I learned that we all have a purpose and a calling in life that we must each discover on our own and in our own time. I will share this and so much more with you. As you continue reading, you will learn and continue to grow spiritually, physically, mentally, emotionally, and psychologically.

After about six months, I decided that it was time to start going out and dating again. Having played the bar scene before, I decided that was no longer for me and if all else failed, would be my last option, so I turned to the Internet. It was amazing...I quickly discovered that there were so many single people in this world! It was mind blowing!

So I began searching through the online personals of many different websites. Because of the vast number of single people available on the Internet, I decided that the very first thing that needed to be done was to set some standards. That is, the females that I wanted to meet had to live in a close proximity of the city I lived in, they had to be between a certain age range, height range, weight range, ethnicity, profession, and looks. All kidding aside, I had a strict set of parameters that I was looking for and did not want to waste my time or anyone else's time in the pursuit of my next date.

To my surprise, I quickly learned that this process of setting standards would pay dividends because I CHOSE to spend my time only talking to women that I felt compatible with. Everyone else was just a waste of my time and money. When the time came for me to actually speak with them either in person or over the phone, I felt sincere and confident and as a result we both ended up having a great time.

All together, I met, dated, and had affairs with seven different women before finally meeting my current wife, Rose. Please do not mistake me for being a player or someone who is bragging. I was just very determined to find the right person and it obviously took me more than one attempt. I cannot take credit for being the best there is on this subject, however I was very persistent.

The first person I met was someone located about 100 miles to the West from where I lived. I did this on purpose because of being concerned about the outcome and not sure what might happen. This way I would not have to worry about being embarrassed or talked about in my local area. As it turns out, she was a very nice person that looked better in her online picture than in person...(no big deal), she had her own house surrounded by beautiful mountains, she was successful in her profession, and we enjoyed each other's company watching TV and going out to dinner.

We did have sex the first night even though I was just testing things out and not sure what the outcome would be. After spending two days with her in her house, we both amicably agreed that there was no lasting spark between us beyond having sex. What a relief it was, because I did not want to hurt her feelings in any way and yet I was not feeling the same attraction in person that I did over the Internet. We are still friends and occasionally send emails to just say hello and see how the other is doing.

The second person I met was someone that lived locally. She looked absolutely gorgeous in her online photo and I just knew this was the person for me. Excited with anticipation to meet her, we decided to meet up at a nice restaurant and have dinner for our first meeting and date. To my surprise, she was about 50 pounds bigger than in her online photo. I would later find out that the photo she used was taken four years earlier. Maintaining my composure and being a gentleman I treated her like a lady and enjoyed having a very nice dinner with her. After dinner we talked for about 30 minutes and being disappointed by the fact she would mislead me that way, I decided that it was time for me go home.

To be quite honest, I was very disappointed because I felt as if I had met one person over the Internet and a completely different person face to face. So the next day I called her up to share my feelings with her and she immediately begin insisting that she wanted to come over to my house and talk to me in person. I reluctantly agreed to let her come over and speak with me in person, thinking this would be my opportunity to let her know that I did not think things were going to work out for us. The challenge with her is that she had this exotic look to her that I found very attractive and in the back of my mind I felt as if she were a very loving and caring person.

When she got to my house later that evening, we sat down to a glass of wine and began talking. She explained to me that she had been abused in past relationships and that she didn't believe in having sex on the first date. I explained that I completely understand and respect her for that. The more we talked and drank wine, the more attracted she became to me physically. Thinking to myself, I can learn to overlook the fact that she is overweight as long as she has a wonderful attitude and great disposition on life.

As the evening progresses, we had a few more glasses of wine, and had gotten to know each other a little better...at least on the surface. She had decided that she wanted to stay and spend the night with me. At this point, I was really torn. Half my brain was telling me that she is a very nice and attractive person and that I could possibly fall in love with her and the other half of my brain was telling me NO DO NOT GET INVOLVED! After debating it over and over in my own mind for about an hour, I finally gave in to her and agreed to let her stay the night.

We had wonderful sex and really seemed to enjoy each other's company. I honestly started feeling as if I could fall in love with this person and enjoy a nice meaningful relationship despite her physical challenges. The next morning after we wake up, she tells me she has to get going because of something going on that day. Feeling a little concerned about her abruptness, I decided to slow things down a little bit. I immediately began to protect myself by controlling my feelings toward her until I felt more comfortable about the whole situation.

Later that evening, she calls me back and wants to come over again and spend the night. I explained to her that I felt that we should take things a little slowly and that it might be best if we did not see each other tonight. Almost immediately, she became a different person and began crying and getting upset and acting as if she had just lost her only friend in the world. At this point I started getting very concerned about who she really was. She insisted on coming over so we could talk some more because there were things about herself that she wanted to share with me.

Being compassionate and caring about her, I let her come back over so we could talk some more. To my surprise, I learn that she has some serious inferiority complexes with herself. So serious that it was to the point where she was contemplating suicide. I was really concerned and listened to all of the problems she was having and offered her some sound objective advice on how to deal with some of her issues. Afterwards, I felt obligated to let her know about my feelings towards her so that I could be there to help her cope with it and prevent her from doing something stupid to herself.

I explained that even though I was attracted to her, I did not feel that she was the right person for me to be involved in a relationship with. She reluctantly accepted this and begged to spend the night with me. Torn again between what to do, I agreed to let her stay the night, at least this way I could ensure that she did not hurt herself. She begged me to make love to her one last time and we both enjoyed the experience. We talked on a daily basis for several weeks after she left and she informed me that the advice I had given her was beginning to help her out and that she was feeling much better about herself.

The third person I met over the Internet was definitely much more in line with what I was looking for. She was close to my age, had been divorced with no kids, had her own house, successful in her career, very optimistic and positive attitude and very confident about herself. This was a welcome relief after the first two experiences. Finally, I met someone that I was compatible with in many ways. We spent three months dating each other, enjoying each others company, making love, and visiting different places together.

After three months, it became the same old routine...week after week. I started feeling like I was married again except this time I never said "I-DO". I found myself feeling as if something was missing in our relationship. She was very attractive, had everything going for her but I still felt something was missing. I needed more spontaneity in my life and was not ready to just settle down again into another same old routine. After explaining to her that I wanted to be able to date other people, she agreed and we were still able to date each other. This lasted for about another three months until I finally decided that I wanted something completely different.

So I logged back on to the online personals and began looking for the fourth person that I was going to meet. At this point, I decided that I was going to meet an Asian woman. Almost immediately I found tons of them from every country over in Asia. I found one in particular that immediately caught my eye. She was very successful, very beautiful, very adventurous, loved to travel, very well educated. What more could I have asked for? I immediately sent her an email and we began chatting online over "AOL Instant Messenger". After about four weeks of chatting and speaking to each other over the phone, she insisted that she has to fly over from Taiwan to meet me and see me in person.

Of course I'm just as anxious to see her and definitely agreed. Two weeks later she arrived at the airport and there I was meeting someone in person for the very first time in my life that I had met online that actually flew half-way around the world from another country just to meet me. I was really excited, anxious, nervous, and scared all at the same time. Up to this point, this is the biggest challenge that I have ever undertaken as far as meeting someone over the Internet. As it turns out, she looked exactly like her photo presented her. She ended up staying for an entire week and we had a great time traveling, watching movies, cooking and getting to know each other.

What really surprised me about her was that she came across as being a very strict virgin and yet made love to me the very first night she arrived and each additional night she stayed with me. I also found out that she was a graduate from Arizona State University and that her religious affiliation was Mormon which was against pre-marital sex, cursing, smoking, and drinking alcohol and caffeine but yet we had sex every night she was here.

When it came time for her to fly back to Taiwan, I escorted her back to the airport and we said our good byes and kept in touch with each other for about two weeks. Then out of the blue she calls me crying saying that she misses me and wants to come see me again. I was surprised because that involved her having to fly all the way from Taiwan again with her out-of-pocket expense for another round-trip ticket costing approx. $1,400.00. This will be the second ticket she purchased in less than two months to come see me.

At this point I felt good about our relationship and with her as a person, so I agreed to let her come back for another week to visit me. This time things were a little different. We still had sex every night but this time she was coming across as being a lot more strict towards me, and started talking about marriage and having children. Immediately I hear brakes screeching to a complete halt in my brain. I thought to myself, I've only known this person for just over two months and she's already making wedding plans and talking about having children!?

At this point, I'm having flashbacks from my first marriage not working out and thinking how much more complicated things would have been if we had had children. So I start thinking to myself that things are going just a little too fast here with Ms. Taiwan and that I better do something quick to slow things down. By this point she was convinced that we were going to get married and I honestly believe she felt that she could start talking to me like she was already my wife. Well needless to say I could see right then and there that this was not going to work out because I did not like what I was seeing or hearing while trying to imagine her being my wife for the rest of my life.

So I decided to play along with her for the remainder of the week until she had to fly back to Taiwan and then I was going to let her know how I was feeling. I did this because for some reason I just wasn't convinced that she would be an easy person to talk to and explain this to in person and that it would be much better to have this conversation with her over the phone. Well needless to say, she was very upset and at this point I had to let her know that I did not want to continue our relationship and expressed my concerns about her strict religious values while simultaneously thinking it was perfectly OK to have pre-marital sex with me. Clearly something just didn't seem right.

So I broke off our relationship and figured it was time for me to take a break for a while from the online dating scene. Well about 2 months later I get a phone call from my ex-online girlfriend in Taiwan informing me that she is pregnant. All I could do was gasp for air and ask her, are you sure? She said she was positive because she had missed her period. Well I'm no dummy when it comes to knowing that just because a woman misses her period, she is pregnant. So I asked if she had gone to see a doctor to confirm her pregnancy and she said that she was planning on it. A few days later I get another call from her telling me that the doctor said that she is pregnant.

I felt as if a ton of bricks had just been placed on my chest. I was confused, upset, and frustrated while thinking, how could I have let this happen to myself? "You Idiot", I thought, "how in the world am I going to deal with this situation"? There was no book written to explain what to do in cases of getting someone pregnant that you met online and lives halfway around the world. So I asked her to go and get a second opinion and she calmly and very willingly agreed.

It was almost as if I could sense a spark of joy coming from her over the phone, while thinking to herself that she was going to end up being with me either way.

Meantime, I'm having one of the most difficult times of my life processing the thought of having a child with someone I really did not feel I was compatible with and who lived over 10,000 miles away. So I started doing some serious praying asking God for help and forgiveness and promising that I would never do this again. You can only imagine that for the next several days I was a complete nervous wreck. Finally, four days later she calls back again to inform me that the second test came back positive as well. Bam! Another blow to my chest! I thought, "how am I going to deal with this"?

So we both talked for about an hour discussing how to handle this situation that we were both in. By the end of our conversation, she told me she had decided to keep the baby and that she realized that it was wrong of her to go against her religious moral and beliefs and to lead me on the way that she did. I explained to her that I was at a complete loss because certainly I wanted to be responsible and do the right thing in fathering my child and at the same time, I wasn't prepared for such responsibility. We were both torn. All I could keep thinking to myself was "what do you do in this type of situation"? It was completely new to me and nobody could advise me because they had never been in this situation before.

Sure I thought about marrying her and even talked to her about the possibility of us getting married but she wanted to stay in Taiwan and I wanted to remain in the U.S. How is that going to work, I thought? So we kept communicating through AOL online chat and called each other as time permitted and she could see how sincere I was in wanting to do the right thing. Well I honestly feel that to this day my sincerity and good nature began getting the best of her because one day, out of the blue, while we were talking on the phone, she told me that she has something very important to tell me.

So immediately I have a thousand thoughts racing through my mind thinking to myself, "What Now"? So she goes on to tell me that she had been keeping a secret from me and that she felt bad because she did not want to hurt me. So naturally being concerned, I blurted out, "what is it"? She begins telling me that she had another affair with someone else when she arrived back in Taiwan after visiting with me and that they had sexual intercourse and that the baby was actually conceived between her and the other person. Well I immediately became infuriated from the thought of having to live with this emotional burden for the previous several months and having every thought you could possibly imagine racing through my mind during that time.

"How could you do this to me"? I asked. Needless to say she felt very bad and I began feeling a tremendous sense of relief. So I informed her that I had nothing else to say to her and wished her good luck with raising her child and let her know that I never wanted to speak with her again for what she had put me through. I hung up and it was over with her. Thank God!

Well at this point I really needed to take a break and decided that I would just enjoy being single for the next six months. Three months had gone by and I was starting to feel lonely again so I began logging back in to Yahoo's online personals and looking to see who else was out there looking for someone. At this point I was still interested in meeting another Asian woman except this time I was going to look for someone already located in the U.S.

I actually found quite a few online personals that met the basics of what I was looking for, so I began sending correspondence to a few of these Asian women. Within a few days I started getting replies and made decision to narrow my focus on two of them. One of them replied back immediately and the other one I never heard from again. So I decide to engage in further communication with the one that replied back. Her online photo and profile portrayed her as being very beautiful, outgoing, adventurous, caring, and loving. Her Asian ethnicity was Pilipino and from what I could see in her photo, she looked very attractive.

Well we continued talking on the phone and chatting online getting to know each other and after about two weeks she pops the big question. "Can I come to Virginia and visit you"? By this point I felt comfortable enough with her and could not think of any problems with having her fly from the West Coast to visit me on the East Coast. So I told her "certainly she could come visit me". Thanksgiving was two weeks away so we made plans for her to fly in to visit me the week of Thanksgiving and we would spend Thanksgiving together. The least expensive last minute flight we could find was flying into BWI which was about a three hour drive for me. Please understand that it was her idea to want to fly and visit so I did not offer to pay for her flight. She willingly paid her own airfare.

So a friend of mine was nice enough and offered to drive me in to BWI to meet her and pick her up so that we could sit in the back seat and talk and get to know each other, and upon seeing her in person for the very first time, I was became extremely embarrassed realizing that she looked totally different in person than from her online photo and began having flashbacks of making the wrong decision again. Apparently she had gained about 40 pounds from the time she left the West Coast and landed on the East Coast because the photos she used in her online profile as well as the photos she had emailed to me showed a very muscular and tone physique, not a 40 pound overweight short Asian girl. Not to mention that in her photos, she had very long beautiful hair and when she landed, she had very short hair.

As she is walking towards me smiling from ear to ear, I'm standing there trying to put on my best face while realizing that I just made another big mistake by allowing someone else to come in to my life that totally misrepresented herself to me. I remember my demeanor going from a happy, joyful person to an immediate state of frustration and I could feel my face turning red from embarrassment. What made things worse is that I shared her photos to all of my friends and was looking forward to introducing her to them. Suddenly, that all changed in the blink of an eye. I remember thinking to myself, "I'm not going to introduce her to any of my friends" in fear of them laughing at me and reminding me of how stupid I was for being so risky.

As it turns out, my friend drove us back to Richmond and I gave her some lame excuse that I wanted to stay home and spend time with her and really get to know her. Little did she know that I CHOSE to make this decision because she totally embarrassed me and completely misrepresented herself, and I was not about to introduce her to my friends and get further embarrassed and certainly was not going to go out painting the town spending money on her. She chose to misrepresent herself so I figured it was my choice on how I wanted to respond and I did.

I so caught off guard and embarrassed that I actually remember wishing that time would just fly by so that I could hurry up and get myself out of this embarrassing situation. So pretty much we stayed at my house the entire time with one exception. While she was there, we did engage in having sex with each other several times and there was a bit of a slight accident and as a result, I had to take her to a clinic to get a morning-after pill. After that incident, I decided that I no longer wanted to be sexually involved with her and I had a heart to heart talk with her explaining how I felt about her misleading me.

She told me that she had misled me because she felt that she would not have had the opportunity to see me otherwise. I conveyed to her how disappointed I was and that I did not want to continue dating her and that there was not going to be a future for us in being together. I know this may sound harsh but one thing you have got to learn from this experience is that if you are going to pursue online dating, you have got to be totally honest with the people you are getting involved with because sooner or later they are going to find out the truth about you. Sooner or later you are going to have to face them.

At this point I had zero tolerance for playing mind games with anyone else. I was so happy after telling her how I felt about what she did and it was such a relief to get that off of my chest and I was really happy when it was time for me to drive her back to BWI airport knowing that she would be out of my life for good. What a relief! The most embarrassing week of my life was over!

This time I was a little more determined to jump right back in to finding someone online and still had my heart set on finding a beautiful Asian woman especially after experiencing such a let down. I remember thinking…"it has got to be better than what I just experienced!"

So there I go again after a few days logging back in and searching for Ms. Right. Almost immediately I discovered a very beautiful Chinese female that had just posted her profile online. I quickly realized that she was over in China. This was good and bad because I would not have to worry about any sudden quick visits that end up disappointing me but at the same time, she was over 10,000 miles away.

We began by just chatting at first and then after about a week I started calling her and talking to her in person. I remember her voice being so soft and beautiful and imagining how beautiful she must be in person. Well this went on for several months and I started to become very interested in wanting to see her. It seemed that this time everything was working out the way I had envisioned it. At least on the surface, or perhaps I was so blind that I did not want to accept anything other than what I wanted to believe.

Well long story short, she ended up mailing me some photos of herself and to me that was confirmation enough for me to want to have her come visit and see how things would go for us. Well at least on the surface it seemed like she had a little bit of an idea of what she wanted to see happen. She was a 23 year old virgin and was not looking for someone to just date and see how things worked out. She was looking for somebody that she could get involved with that was going to marry her and bring her over to the U.S. and start a family. That was all fine and well except I was determined that there was no way in this world that I was going to have any kids. It just wasn't in the plans.

After a few months, we both realized that we were very attracted to each other and that the chemistry was definitely there, but that we were both looking for different outcomes. In realizing this, we both agreed to not pursue furthering our relationship with each other. It was a very sad time for both of us because the chemistry was definitely present between us. Had I wanted to have children at that time, she would have been the ideal wife for me, but that was not in the cards at this time. We slowly stopped sending each other emails and chatting and eventually she just faded in to the past and I never heard from her again, which brings me to lucky number seven, my wife and life partner.

Please understand that at this point I was striking out with every attempt and had pretty much decided to give up! And wouldn't you know it...just as with every great story in life, there is always a turning point. So after allowing 4 months to pass by and giving up on the idea that I would find that perfect someone through the internet that I could spend the rest of my life with, I suddenly had an epiphany!

The epiphany was when I decided to date someone that came to work at my office as a temp. She was all American and from the outside she looked very beautiful and desirable. From the inside, she was just the opposite. She was very mean spirited, had a lot of baggage, already had a child, and was a single mother with a bad attitude that would never shut up. I mean she would not stop talking! As soon as she realized that I was interested in dating her, she immediately began putting on a fake front when she was around me.

It was not until after we had dated several times that I really saw her true colors and experienced my epiphany. Some very close friends of mine invited me out for dinner with them at a very nice restaurant and I accepted the offer. Since my friends were all married and going as couples, I invited my (then) girlfriend to go with me as my date and she immediately accepted. While at dinner, we were all having drinks and laughing and having fun and I specifically remember my date just rambling on and on about any and everything and being very negative about this and about that.

You have to imagine for a minute that she is one of these people who would always have something negative to say about whatever topic you might be talking about. No matter how great or grand the outcome really is, she has something negative to say and does not know how to keep her mouth shut. Well about halfway through our evening she opens her big mouth and makes a comment about me to my friends by saying something very negative. My friends know me very well and realize at this point what type of person she really is and just kind of laugh it off knowing that what she just said was not true.

Well I just sat there and pretty much kept quiet for the rest of the evening minding my own business and casually talking to my friends and ignoring my girlfriend until it was time to go. We go ahead and pay the bill and leave and I'm taking my girlfriend back to my house, where her car is parked. The plan was that she was going to spend the night with me and go pick up her son in the morning. At this point she had had just a little too much to drink and just would not shut up at all. Meanwhile, I'm just biting my tongue listening to her and trying not to get engaged in conversation with her.

Right as I pull up in my driveway, she made a very negative comment about one of my friends that we just had dinner with and at that point I decided that I had had enough of her. I stopped the car told her that she needed to learn to shut her mouth and that she needed to get in her car and go home because I did not want her to spend the night and did not want to date her anymore. It was at that point that I had my epiphany and decided that as soon as I got in my house, I was going to log back on to the internet and immediately start looking for my ideal wife.

This time it was going to be different because by this point I knew exactly who I wanted to meet and what I was looking for in the ideal person. After having gone through so much adversity and constant challenges in trying to find Ms. Right, I knew exactly what I wanted in the ideal person down to the ethnic background, the personality, the type of work they did, and the exact industry I wanted them to be involved in.

Please understand the importance here! The time and effort it took me to reach my epiphany did not happen over night. As you just read in the previous pages, I had to make a lot of mistakes to finally get to the point to realize that if I wanted this "internet-dating" thing to work out for me, **I had to figure out exactly what I wanted in the ideal person first, and then focus all my attention on finding this person.** As it turned out, this proved to be 90% of my challenges in finding the right person. Too many people that I talk to keep telling me over and over that they are just looking for someone that they are compatible with and can get along with. Well I hate to be the bearer of bad news but that just is not going to cut it. That is way too vague!

The Big Secret in this is that you have got to get very specific about who you want to meet, what you want them to look and feel like, what ethnic background you want them to be from, what type of personality they need to have, what type of work they do, and specifically what you want and expect out of the relationship.

The more specific you and your expectations are the better your chances are of finding the right person. If you are not prepared to be specific with the details about who you are looking for, then you are going to waste a lot of your time and money and possibly someone else's, spinning your wheels like I did and not make any progress. Remember, **"we become what we think about and move in the direction of our most dominant thought"**...more on this later in the book!

I knew specifically that I wanted my next wife (the person I wanted to spend the rest of my life with) to be Asian, beautiful, knows how to cook, has a great attitude, was good in sales, and involved in the Information Technology industry, and was very independent! I realized after years of experience of falling for whatever came my way how important these specific qualities were in the next person that I was going to be committed to for the rest of my life! I finally got it!! Until I found the person with the qualities I was looking for...I would never be truly happy in my relationships. I knew myself well enough to realize that I would keep looking for my "Ms. Right" even if it meant cheating until I found those qualities in someone.

So for me that was it! I was ready to make my commitment and set out to find the lady of my dreams! I was so focused on the exact type of person that I wanted to meet, that I knew it inside and out and immediately I felt this calm sense of knowing that I would find her, it was just a matter of time. Once I knew exactly what characteristics I wanted in this ideal person, I narrowed my focus and set out with my parameters and found her! She met and exceeded every expectation that I set for myself (you can see a picture of us and our beautiful daughter on the back cover of this book). You have got to be focused like a laser beam! You know the old saying..."if you do not stand for something, you will fall for anything". It's amazing once you know exactly what you are looking for, how quickly you can find it!

So going forward, know exactly what type of person you are looking for and focus all of your time and attention on finding them, otherwise you will end up falling for whatever comes along and you will soon realize that you still have that unfulfilled feeling inside of you. So get focused, be specific, have patience, have faith in the fact that you will find the right person in good time, stay positive, and be flexible and in the meantime, learn the important lessons in this book to better understand how to prepare yourself to seize your opportunity when it approaches! Just as importantly, keep visualizing in your mind the day you meet the person of your dreams and now start preparing yourself for that moment!

Good Luck and Success to you and all of your relationships from this moment forward! I hope that you enjoy learning the valuable lessons in this book and continue applying them to all of your relationships for the rest of your new life. Your best approach may be to take one lesson per day and read and focus on that one lesson. The next day, read and focus on the next topic, and so on. This will help you learn and metabolize each valuable topic and soon you will be full of the kind of knowledge needed to have very successful relationships in all aspects of your life! Congratulations on your decision to begin improving your existing relationships and discovering new ones...now let us get to work on learning some more important information!

Chapter 2:

"Psychological Factors To Consider
Before Looking For New Relationships"

Before setting your heart on meeting, greeting and embracing new people through the Internet, the Grocery Store, the Mall, or wherever, it is extremely important that you first take some important psychological factors into consideration about dating and human beings that you can begin applying and using from this moment forward that will help you in all of your relationships. These psychological factors pertain to relationships with your family, co-workers, old friends, new friends, your spouse, your lovers...pretty much everyone that you have to interact with.

Please keep in mind that the lessons laid out over the next 73 chapters that you are about to learn are like a two-edged sword. Meaning that just as you will learn to listen, identify, and look out for certain things that are happening in your relationships that may be causing problems, you need to also make sure that YOU are not the person causing these problems in the relationship and I will show you how you can identify and make sure of that later in this book.

Please keep in mind that these lessons will consist of words, phrases and advice that you will want to become aware of and learn to listen out for whenever you engage in conversation with any of your relationships from this moment forward. I really wish someone had put this valuable information in front of me when I was about 20 years old because it sure would have made a big difference in all of my relationships along the way.

Please refer back to these lessons often so you can to continue learning how to improve your relationships. For each time you re-read them, you will learn something new and unique that you may not have noticed the first time you read them. Again, congratulations on taking a very positive step forward on improving all of your relationships!

Chapter 3:

"Relationships"

Relationships - Every relationship and especially marriage takes an ongoing daily effort from each person involved. A lot of people think or feel that once they have found their "Mr. or Ms. Right", they can kick back, relax, take it easy, and enjoy life happily ever after. Well that might sound great if you are living in a fairy tale somewhere far, far away. But, I hate to be the bearer of bad news because that type of behavior does not apply nor work in human relationships. Thus, we introduce the concept called "The Human Factor". At least this is what I have titled this factor as for the purposes of this book.

"The Human Factor" is a relationship factor that one must be aware of at all times, must be included into the relationship equation, and yet has no rhyme or reason. The only way of possibly including "The Human Factor" into your relationships is to simply be aware that it really does exist and by constantly being aware of and adjusting your feelings, philosophies, moods, emotions, words, thoughts, and actions accordingly to the person you are involved with or about to get involved with and can have a huge impact on the outcome of your relationship(s).

Simply put, every human being has their own set of ideals, beliefs, philosophies, prejudices, tolerance level, and understanding of how things are supposed to be. Amazingly, no two individuals' beliefs and life-concepts are the same. Therefore, you must be aware of this when deciding to enter into any relationship and be able to adjust yourself according to the other person's beliefs and vice versa if the relationship is going to have any lasting success.

Just because we are finally married or dating someone steadily does not mean that we have the privilege of no longer having to work on improving our relationship by adapting, adjusting, and factoring in the other persons wants and needs and expectations. In fact just the opposite is true. As more time passes in our relationships, the harder we have to work at keeping them balanced because of more responsibilities being placed upon us as the relationship progresses and having less time for ourselves. Therefore, we have to continue working diligently every single day on maintaining and improving our relationship just as we would expect from all of our relationship partners...this applies whether they are your friend, family, lover, or foe!

This can only be accomplished through down-to-earth honest and open communication, patience, forgiveness, participation, initiation, acceptance, and persistence. The ideal loving relationship would consist of two individuals that intellectually, mentally, and physically are stimulating to each other which helps keep their relationship vibrant and interesting. These two need to be respectful, caring, understanding and supportive of one another through good times and bad. An open line of communication is an absolute must if the relationship is going to continue being strong through good times and bad!

In addition to continually working on improving your communication skills, each partner should also want to keep themselves in good health, hygiene, and physical condition, both for their own benefits and to help their significant other continue to remain interested in them. Many times, I meet people who have been together for several years or more and I have noticed that they have started to either gain a lot of weight, or stopped working out, or let their hygiene go downhill or began treating their significant other without respect. When I see this, I think to myself, it is just a matter of time before the other person decides they have had enough of this relationship, or meets someone new that they find attractive, and fulfilling to their own needs in their desired relationship, and perhaps sees that this new person is keeping them self in a much better shape and health condition that is more conducive to their expectations, and that they will eventually fall for if given enough time and tension in the current relationship.

The rule of thumb that we should learn to follow is that we should never allow ourselves to become complacent in our relationships, and should always strive to make our relationships better and more enjoyable every single day that we are involved in them. After all, the definition of success is "the favorable or prosperous termination of attempts or endeavors". Keep focusing and thinking every day about how successful you would like to see your relationship(s) become and to what level. By doing so, you will be more inclined to conduct yourself in such a way as to bring out the desired end result. After you have achieved your desired end result, keep working on maintaining and making that relationship even better and add in some humor and confidence and the person you are involved with will find it very difficult to ever want to consider leaving you.

So remember, when you find yourself with the perfect person or involved in the ideal relationship, keep pressing forward every single day to improve your relationship as well as yourself, your health, and your personal hygiene and notice how your loving relationships will want to continue staying with you and in return will feel motivated by you being so proactive about taking good care of yourself, that they will want to do the same by taking good care of them self. At this point you have a very balanced, open-communication relationship that continually motivates each other to be a better person. When you get to this point, it is next to impossible to not continually feel in love with your partner and vice-versa and there is a very positive understanding and energy between both of you.

However, on the flip side, if only one partner is striving to continually better them self and doing things to keep the relationship strong and vibrant and the other partner is not, then the relationship will not be balanced and eventually a change will have to be made to balance out the relationship, one way or another.

Chapter 4:

"Communication"

Communication - Believe it or not, open and effective communication can carry a relationship through the toughest of times and bring people closer together at the same time. However, lack of open and effective communication can become the number one cause for most problems in relationships and marriages. Think about it! Why do most people end up arguing? Most people end up arguing because of lack of understanding or lack of effective communication in their relationships. Usually this happens because one person in the relationship is concerned or is in fear of the other person finding out something that they may not like or approve of so they suppress the information or create diversions to avoid having to talk about or face the real issues.

Instead of facing their fears by openly talking to their partner and addressing these hidden concerned issues right from the very beginning, they continue to cover them up and deny and create fabrications in an attempt to avoid talking about whatever the real issue is. The best way to handle these types of situations is to bring issues and/or concerns out into the open in the form of a calm discussion explaining to your partner that you absolutely love and respect them and that there are some things you want to get out into the open because sooner or later they will be found out. Explain that you would rather be open and honest and tell them right now than try to pretend that these issues or concerns do not exist and cover them up only to be found out later.

The reality is that if this person you are involved with really and truly loves you and sincerely cares for you, they will either be understanding and find a way to work with you around your issues or concerns or in so many words, they will tell you that this is not a relationship they want to continue being involved in. Either way, it is better to be upfront and honest and know that the person you are involved with knows and understands who you really are and loves you for who you are, than to purposely avert the inevitable truth and live in constant fear that some day they are going to find out the truth about you and be really upset because you did not properly and openly communicate with them in an honest way.

The underlying reasons why people act in this type of behavior stem directly either from their ego, low self esteem, feelings of rejection, and/or fear of loss. All of this points directly to your ego because nobody likes to have their feelings hurt, or be rejected, and feelings are a direct correlation to your ego or feeling of self-importance. Most people will go out of their way and do some pretty crazy things in a vain attempt to protect their feelings of self-importance or ego. The best answer however, is to literally "set your ego aside", humble yourself, suck it up, and deal with whatever the consequences are going to be at that moment and not allowing the end result to devastate you if it is not what you were expecting the outcome to be.

This is called doing the right thing and being true to yourself, and you will be able to sleep better at night knowing that you did the right thing by effectively communicating. Besides, I would much rather be true to myself and sleep good at night, than live in fear or a bubble of make-believe because I was so consumed with my own ego and did not effectively communicate and tell the truth. Just like building a house, your relationship will be based on a solid foundation or a deck of cards. How YOU CHOOSE to communicate will determine the strength of your relationship foundation.

The examples I have given can be summed up and viewed as a lack of open-communication, a lack of miscommunication, or just an outright deliberate decision to not communicate for one reason or another. However you slice it, it is still a form of Lack of Communication and it is an issue that needs to be dealt with immediately before any relationship can be expected to improve or get any better. Until the level of quality and honest communication does get better, the relationship will only continue to stagnate and sour and eventually become unmanageable.

I know this because I have experienced it personally. How many times have you caught yourself or someone else saying..."you just don't understand me", or "you never pay attention to what I am saying"? Have you ever thought that maybe it is because you do not know how to properly communicate with your partner or vice-versa? Could it be that one of you is not properly communicating the whole truth because there are some underlying issues or an ego getting in the way? Whatever the reason, it must be dealt with before the relationship between both of you can improve and continue moving on the right track. Learn to openly and honestly communicate and get past your problems to get back on track to the fun and loving relationship that you were ultimately after.

So what exactly is proper communication and why does it play such an important role in relationships? Communication is the ability to openly and honestly convey and express your feelings, thoughts and emotions about what is important to you on the inside and the outside to another individual that is ready, willing and able to listen. Ideal communication is when you and your significant other can take turns conveying your feelings and emotions openly and honestly without conditions to each other while the other is willing to quietly sit and attentively listen with concern, understanding and compassion.

Communication plays such an important role in relationships because it is the only universal vehicle that we as humans have to explain how we think, feel, and want to be treated. It is the passageway for our feelings and emotions to be conveyed from one individual to another. Ideal Communication allows us to talk about the problems we feel we have and be able to share that which bothers us inside whether it would be feelings of love, frustration, jealousy, envy, hate, resentment etc. Communication also allows us to clear out the ill-feelings we have bottled up inside so we do not explode or implode psychologically or emotionally.

Effective communication can make us feel calm, soothed, loved, respected, understood, and appreciated. The strongest man in the world could probably lift 1,000 pounds and yet have bottled up emotions which have no physical weight that could literally crush his character and being. Most people that break up because of having money problems in their relationship break up mostly because of their lack of communication and understanding about the money problems rather than the money problem itself.

Think about it! Most people would say that money problems are the major cause for problems in relationships. I have to disagree because the money problems can be resolved over a period of time if proper communication and understanding are in order. However the smallest perceived problems in a relationship can become extremely difficult to solve if the communication and understanding are not in order. You can have all of the money in the world and not be an effective communicator and have a lot of relationship problems. Trust me I have experienced both sides first-hand. A lack of communication can literally break up a seemingly wonderful relationship in a matter of days. So CHOOSE to continue to learn to be an effective and good communicator.

A good communicator is not just someone who knows how to talk. A good communicator consist more of someone who knows how to listen attentively with sincere genuineness and understanding. A good communicator allows the person speaking to completely say what is on their mind without interruption or judgment. One of the best rules you can begin to establish to become a great communicator is called the **"3 second rule"**. The **"3 second rule"** is simply counting One-thousand-one, One-thousand-two, One-thousand-three after someone finishes speaking and before you begin speaking or replying back to them.

You do this for several good reasons.

1. It shows the person who is speaking to you that you are more concerned with what they are saying than with what you have to say to them in response.

2. It also shows the person speaking that you respect them by not immediately responding the moment they stop speaking or pause for a breath and allows the conversation to be calm and productive.

3. It also conveys the message to the person speaking that you are genuinely interested in them demonstrated through your attentiveness, and as a result of our human nature, the speaker will begin to like you even more for taking the time to listen to them.

So the next time you find yourself involved in a conversation remember to CHOOSE to be a good listener and give the person speaking your undivided attention. They will be sure to like you much more as a result and because of the law of psychological reciprocity, they will return the same respect to you when it is time for you to speak. If someone seems to be dominating the conversation and you need to get to an appointment, simply say to them..."excuse me, I have got an appointment to get to in 30 minutes and I really want to continue our conversation, when can you be available so we can continue this conversation later this evening or tomorrow?

Also, when you are on a date with someone for the first time and you notice that they are dominating the conversation, as long as you feel comfortable with letting them dominate the conversation, let them continue. If you begin to feel that they are talking way too much and it is not an interesting or important conversation, simply say to them in a very polite way..."excuse me, you know I have had a very long day today and I was wondering if you and I could pick up this conversation at a later time so that you and I can enjoy this beautiful quiet evening together over a glass of wine or dinner? They will get the hint and then they will start focusing in on you more. After the date is over, you will then need to decide if this is the right person for you or not.

If you feel that they are not the right person for you thank them for a great evening and be honest and upfront with them. Be nice about it and yet be honest with them and yourself. Remember it is YOUR CHOICE! Do not play games or try to avoid them. That only delays the inevitable and might cause you to have a bad reputation. Simply tell them..."for whatever reason, I just do not feel the type of bond that I am looking for in a relationship between us. I know that you deserve someone very special and I would like to know if we could continue to just be friends?" If they say sure, then you have met a new friend for life, if they say no, then you definitely made the right decision. Either way, your effective communication skills have allowed you to win and continue to move forward without hurting anyone or pinning yourself into a corner.

Most importantly, take responsibility for making sure that YOU are being understood and that YOU understand what the other person is saying. You do this by politely asking for clarification in a non-threatening or non-demeaning way. For Example: "So let me make sure I fully understand what you are telling me, what you are saying is that......bla, bla, bla, is that correct?" Conversely, it is just as important to make sure that you take the responsibility for making sure that the other person understands what you are saying. For Example: "What I mean by that, is that.....bla, bla, bla, is that OK with you?" Ask for clarification to make sure the other person completely understands what you are saying, and what you meant by what you are saying. So from now on, YOU CHOOSE to be a more effective communicator and watch your relationships become more meaningful as a result.

Chapter 5:

"TRY"

Try – The word "Try" implies failure. You either "Do" or you "Do Not" do something. There is no in between. A lot of people will use the word "Try" as a way of avoiding commitment or to get out of doing something, and most unsuspecting people will fall victim to the use of the word "Try" every time and do not realize what just happened. For example, you may recall being involved in a conversation at some point in your life with someone and recall them saying something like... "I will try to make it there", or "I will try to meet you at 3:00PM", or "I will try to be there to help you"

The very first thing you should do when you hear the word 'try" is stop and realize that what is really being said to you, in so many words, and usually not intended to not hurt your feelings, is that they are not going to be there at all or that they are not going to help you. By taking a deeper look, you may find that the people in your life that constantly use the word "Try" are either insecure with themselves or about themselves and/or they use the word "Try" as a result of a habit that developed early on in their life learned from someone else in their life also using the word "Try".

Either way, excessive use of the word "Try" implies that the individual is attempting to say "No" to you without feeling like they have hurt your feelings by saying "No' or perhaps they do not feel secure enough about themselves to just stand up and say "No" to you because they are concerned about what you might think or feel about them for saying "No" to you. So using the word "Try" is their way of escaping your feelings of discontent towards them and simultaneously allows them to escape from following through with any commitments to you. Think about it! An emotionally secure person will tell you straight up, "NO!", "I cannot help you or be there at that time to help you". They will not lead you to believe that they will be there and then not show up by using the word "Try".

So learn to recognize that most often when someone uses the word "Try", after you have asked them for some type of commitment, that should be a clear indication to you that they most likely will not be there to live up to the commitment and you need to immediately recognize this and make a CHOICE to not be upset with them for not following through with YOUR expected commitment from them.

If their continual use of the word "Try" is presenting a problem for you, then what you have got to do is immediately recognize that what they are really saying to you by using the word "Try" really means "NO" and ask them for a stronger level of commitment. For example, you could say "You know John, rather than trying to meet me at 3:00PM, can you be sure to meet me at 4:00PM?" or "Jill, rather than trying to meet me on Wednesday, can you be certain to meet me on Thursday?" You get the idea, go back and ask for confirmation using an alternative time, day, event etc.

This will come back to you 10 fold in the form of fewer disappointments, more productive time, less stress, and stronger friendships. Please keep in mind that most people do not realize what "Try" really means, nor the effects it can have on relationships. Remember, most people that use the word "Try", will see it as a nice way of saying "NO" or "Not At This Time" to you not realizing the impact it can have on you. So learn to recognize this and the next time you hear the word "try", you will now be that much wiser and better prepared to deal with what someone really means or is really saying to you, so you can begin to CHOOSE to move past this disappointment.

Chapter 6:

"Can't"

Can't – The word "Can't" simply implies that "you either honestly don't know how to do something" or "you just don't want to do something", PERIOD! Most of the time, the word "can't" is used because someone DOES NOT want to do something. Therefore they will use the word "can't" as their scapegoat to get out of doing something and most unsuspecting people will just accept their use of the word "can't" as "not able to" and never question it. "Can't" does not mean "not able to", again, "can't" only means one of two things...either "don't know how to", or "don't want to".

If you do not know how to do something, chances are very good that I can teach you, which means that after I teach you how to do something that you previously said you "can't", you can no longer say that "you do not know how to", now it is a matter of "do you really want to". If you really do not want to do something, then that is really what you meant to say in the beginning when you used the word "can't".

Be careful to listen closely to what people are telling you in your conversations. If they say the word "can't", you should immediately ask yourself, does this mean they "do not know how to" or "do not want to"? If you are not certain, simply ask them, "if I show you how to do this or that", could you help me with the project then? If they say "NO", then immediately recognize that is what they really meant to say from the beginning.

Chapter 7:

"But"

But – The word "But" is a very powerful three-letter word because it negates everything that was said before it. For example: "I really like you...but!" Or, "Everything is going great between us...but!" Or, "I'd love to marry you...but!" Or, "I really would like to go out on a date with you...but!" What is really happening here is that the word "but" is being used as a way to allow the speaker to first say something nice to you and then say what they really think or feel about you or have on their mind.

In fact, as a society we have grown so accustomed to hearing the word "but", that we have evolved to a point whereby we are actually expecting to hear the word "but" in our day-to-day conversations without fail. You hear people all the time beginning to finish another persons sentence, after being told something good or positive by the other person, and actually saying it with emphasis, "**but**", almost as if they are expecting the person speaking to them to have the very next word coming out of their mouth to be something negative. Using the word "but" is now socially acceptable to serve as a transition from saying something positive to saying something negative all in the same sentence.

Remember, whatever comes after the word "but" is what was really meant to be said. I cannot think of one person that anticipates or likes hearing the word "but", because they know that the very next thing said after the word "but" usually equals something negative or bad news. This includes people that you engage in conversations with as well. They know that if you start to say something positive to them, there is a very strong possibility that you are going to throw your big old "but" in the conversation and either say something negative or tell them some bad news that will end up taking away all of the positive feelings you had just given them prior to your using the word "but".

So from now, in place of the word "but", you should start using the word "and". You do this for several good reasons. 1. It forces you to stop and carefully think about what you are about to CHOOSE to say because you have to incorporate the word "and" instead of "but". 2. Using the word "and" in place of "but" keeps everything positive and allows you to convey some additional insight for the other persons benefit on how to make things better in a positive manner without leaving any ill feelings towards you.

Take a look at the following examples of using the word "and" versus "but". "I really like you "but" I don't think we communicate with each other very well." Versus "I really like you "and" I think that if we can work on improving our communication skills, we could have a very open and beautiful relationship." Another example is, "I really would like to date you, "but" I'm just not sure if you are the best candidate for me." Versus "I really would like to date you "and" if I could have a couple of days to make a final decision on who the best candidate is for me, I will be sure to get back in touch with you and let you know." Another example is, "I think we have a good chance at winning the game, "but" if we don't practice more, we are going to loose for sure." Versus, "I think we have a good chance at winning the game "and" if we put in some extra practice time, we stand a chance at also winning the championship."

Can you begin to see how this three letter word can have a big impact on your time, energy and money? Now think of the impact that identifying and eliminating the use of all three words you just learned over the last several pages will start to have in your life. That is, learning to identify and eliminating the words "try", "can't", and "but". So from this moment on, learn to recognize them in your conversations and notice how often you use them as well as how often other people use them in conversations with you and just as importantly, learn to recognize what other people are really telling you with their use of these words.

Once you recognize that you are about to use one of these three words, stop for a moment, think about what you are about to say and what you really want to convey and/or accomplish as the end result. Do you want to let someone down, or build them up? The use of these three words, or lack of use of these three words can and will do just that. At the same time, notice how other people are using these three words in their conversations with you and what they are really meaning to say. You will notice it starts to make a big difference in your understanding of conversations with other people.

Chapter 8:

"Small Commitments"

Small Commitments – Whether you realize this or not, "Small Commitments" lead up to larger commitments. This applies to dating, business, friendships, marriage...you name it. The reason that the understanding of this is so important is because you may not necessarily always get what you are going after at first. So you have to learn to keep you composure, accept what you can get and steadily work towards achieving your goal.

For example, when you meet someone new for the very first time, you do not ask them to give you their inner-most personal secrets, savings account balance, and annual income or marriage. You ask for small commitments at first like, where do you work, what type of restaurants do you like to eat at, what's your favorite sport, do you like to dance, do you have any pets, do you have any family close by etc. etc., and build on this. These are all forms of small commitments.

On your first date, keep it at this pace. People feel comfortable answering questions that are easy for them to answer and that do not require a lot of thought or concern for loss of privacy. Additionally, if they begin answering these small little questions without hesitation, they are already sending signals of showing interest in you and setting the stage for the evolution of larger commitments. Now of course you do not want to make them feel like they are being grilled so be reasonable, take your time, and pace yourself. The key here is to relax and have fun getting to know each other. Make it enjoyable for them to answer your questions.

Understanding how small commitments leads to larger commitments means that sometimes, you have to start with what you can get and work from there. For example: You might want to end up marrying someone special that you found through the Internet or at the grocery store and started dating. However, the other person may want to just take things slowly for awhile and see where it goes from there.

By being patient and realizing that small commitments lead up to larger commitments, you could very well end up marrying that special someone that you have met simply by starting off the relationship with small commitments and gradually leading up to larger commitments over a period of time. The key is to keep a stead progression going with the development and evolution of the relationship. Mix in some humor, confidence, and romantic dates and you have a winning combination going for you.

It does not always happen this way and the important thing to keep in mind here is to keep the thought in the back of your mind that since small commitments do lead to larger commitments, you might want to give that special someone a little space and / or time if your gut feeling is telling you they need it. By doing so, they will recognize that you are not a pushy, clingy, or overbearing high maintenance person and may actually become more attracted to you as a result. The key is gradual nudges in the direction that you ultimately want to move in.

Remember the old saying..."Some is better than none" or "A bird in hand is better than two in the bush" or "I'd rather have a little bit of something than a whole lot of nothing"? Well the same rule applies here except that with this understanding, you can start off with just a little and work your way towards getting a lot in a relatively short time frame. So learn to be patient yet pleasantly persistent and take things in moderation not full speed ahead.

Another example: Let us say you meet and begin to date someone that you really, really like and they tell you that they want to date other people until they can decide who they really want to be with. In most cases, by being patient and understanding towards their needs and concerns, means that you could end up being the person that they want to end up being with. By using continuous gradual nudges that lets this person know how much you really care for them, slowly reinforces the bond and the desire to want to be with you.

Look at this way, by realizing that at least you get to go out with this person and date them, you still win. If you like this person enough, then the challenge you are going to be faced with is if you have enough strength and determination to continue dating this person under these circumstances realizing that they could decide to end up wanting to be with someone else. The key here is to control your emotions and continue to let this person know how much you really care for them through continuous gradual nudges, or as I like to say, be "pleasantly persistent".

In most cases, human nature dictates that the person who really likes you the most and is willing to stay committed to you through good times and bad is the person that you will ultimately end up being with. This of course is provided that there is some form of attraction from each other and towards each other in the first place. So whatever situation you find yourself in, remember, small commitments lead to larger commitments and with this new found knowledge, proceed slowly.

Chapter 9:

"It's NOT What You Say...It's HOW You Say It"

It's Not What You Say, It's How You Say It – We have all heard the old cliché that "It's not what you say, it's how you say it", right? Well this is so true...especially when it comes to communicating with someone that you have a lot of interest in and want to date. I have blown this one so many times that I have stopped counting. And I should be the first person to remember it. Did you realize you could literally tell someone off and use curse words and depending on how you say it, they will think you just joking with them and will not take offense to it.

On the other hand, you can put anger and resentment behind the most beautiful words in the world and you will soon start making enemies. Take the following phrase and do this as an experiment to see first-hand. Say..."I think you are so stupid". Now look in the mirror and practice saying it with a smile and then say it with a serious look on your face. You can almost feel the drastic change in tone and demeanor just by saying the same thing two different ways.

Therefore, it is extremely important to always know what your demeanor is when you are using words or phrases that could have more than one meaning. Practice this next step and see if it works for you. Take the phrase..."Leave me alone" At first say it with a happy smiling face, next along with a smiling face, make your tone a little higher and say it quickly while smiling. Next, say it without smiling, lower your tone, and slow down and emphasize each word. See the difference? It is the same three words, and it is how you say them that matters most. So the next time you go to say something, remember how you want it to come across and be perceived.

Chapter 10:

"Obviously You Have A Reason"

Obviously You Have A Reason – Obviously you have a reason for saying that, do you mind if I ask what it is? One of the most frustrating situations a human being can encounter is being rejected. What makes it even worse, is not knowing why you were rejected, with the possibility that you could correct the problem if you only knew what the problem was. It is kind of like a catch-20.

The best way to go about finding out the real reason that you were rejected is to simply ask. I have learned that the best way to ask someone for that reason is by asking them in a very straight-forward way without making them feel uncomfortable. For Example: Let us say that you meet someone over the Internet and they agree to an initial in-person introduction.

However, once they meet you in person, their perception of who you are, is completely different from who you really are. They will either tell you they are not interested with words or with body language. If you begin to notice or sense that they are not really that interested in you after all, you may want to take the initiative and let them know what you sense or feel about them towards you and simply ask "Do I meet all of the expectations that you are looking for?"

They will either say "of course" or "not really" or something similar. Depending on their enthusiasm, their answer should let you know if they are sincere or just lip-sinking it. If they say "not really", you should calmly reply back with "Obviously, you have a reason for saying that, do you mind if I ask what it is?" They will either begin telling you what the reason is or they will grant you permission to ask them from the question you just asked them "...do you mind if I ask what it is?" In which case go ahead and ask them "What is it about me that does not meet all of your expectations?" Keep quiet and let them answer without you interrupting. This is your chance to learn what other people might see in you that you do not see in yourself.

Chapter 11:

Just Suppose For A Moment – I found out that most people will only tell you part of the reason they make a certain decision and that the only way to uncover all of the reasons (if there are more than one) is to keep asking. After all, this is your opportunity to critique yourself by looking through the eyes of someone else so take full advantage of it while you can.

The best way to uncover and learn if there are more reasons for a certain decision is by simply asking…"Just suppose for a moment that wasn't the issue, then in your opinion do you feel that we would be able to date each other?" What this does is isolate each problem one by one and letting you know if there are more problems that you need to focus on resolving. They will either answer "No" or "Yes". If they answer "No", you should calmly say to them…"Obviously, you have a reason for saying that, do you mind if I ask what it is?". Keep doing this until you uncover all of the possible problems that the other person may see in you that is keeping them from wanting to date you.

You see, the only way you could ever begin to correct or fix a problem is by first knowing what the problem really is. Then once you know what the problem is, you have to make a decision whether you want to correct it or not as talked about in lesson referencing the word "Cannot".

Chapter 12:

"May I Ask Why"

May I Ask Why – I learned back in 1994 that a simple little four word question could really do wonders. I have personally tested this approach well over 1,000 times with great results in various aspects of my life, so I really know how well this works. Depending on your voice inflection, most people will give you a very honest response. Imagine for a moment, that you are in a grocery store and see someone very attractive that you would like to ask out on a date. You proceed closer and begin to introduce yourself and get through some small talk. Suddenly the moment arrives that you have to make a decision to either ask them out on a date or tell them it was nice meeting them and continue shopping.

You proceed to ask them out (using one of the many effective ways I share with you throughout this book) and they decline to accept your offer to go out on a date. At this point, you have already been rejected, so accept it and move on to the next phase, which is learning WHY you were rejected. Take a big deep breath, smile and calmly ask them..."May I ask why?" and remain completely silent while looking right into their eyes and still smiling. 99% of the time, they will tell you the truth if you asked them in a non-threatening and sincere way.

The response could be..."I am already dating someone", "I am only here visiting", "I am going through a divorce or separation", "I am not from this part of town" or whatever the response is. If it comes across as a sincere response and you do not feel uncomfortable with their answer, you could take it one step further by asking them the question from the Lesson: *"Just suppose for a moment that was not a concern, then in your opinion do you feel that we could go out on a date just to get to know each other?"* By doing this, you can really begin to identify and understand what other people see in you and think about you objectively.

The key here is to always remain calm and speak softly so as to not give the impression that you are upset or feel frustrated inside. Rather you want to convey an impression of confidence and assurance in yourself by being cool, calm and collective. Otherwise, they might just walk away and ignore you. Now once you get in your vehicle and the windows are rolled up, then you can scream and yell and let out your frustration. The key here is to get to the real reason why someone would not have gone out on a date with you.

So the next time you get rejected or turned down for a date, remember to quickly, Stop, Keep your composure, Smile, Look the other person in the eye, and ask "May I Ask Why". If you begin to notice a pattern for the reasons you are being turned down, then obviously you need to work on improving that area of your life. You will never know unless you ask WHY.

Chapter 13:

"Body Language"

Body Language – Body Language can tell an awful lot about someone, especially if it is the first time you are meeting them. Of course you have to take in consideration that they may be a little nervous at first. Beyond that though, there are certain things that you will need to look out for and be aware of what they mean.

For example, if you agree to meet someone for the first time to go out on a date and while out on the date, this person keeps looking around and constantly staring at other people while you are having a conversation with them, you should immediately understand that this person is either bored or has something in mind. This may not necessarily mean they are bored with you. It could mean they are bored with what you are talking about.

The best thing to do here is to get them involved in the conversation by asking small little questions that will be easy for them to answer. Hence, small commitments leading to larger commitments. If on the other hand, the person keeps yawning and has a glazed over look on their face, they are definitely bored. You need to quickly find something to do to spice things up a bit. Either go for a nice walk, get up and go dancing, skip rocks across the pond, pick flowers, or something. Whatever you do, don't just keep sitting there knowing this person is bored out of their mind or you may not get a second chance at dating them because they will view you as being too boring.

Chapter 14:

"Honesty"

Honesty – Believe it or not, Honesty still is the best policy. Being true to yourself and how you present yourself to other people allows you to relax and actually just be yourself while around other people and especially when you first start dating someone. Think of it this way, eventually people are going to find out who you really are, it is just a matter of time. So why not put your best honest foot forward to start with? By doing so, you will be able to avoid a lot of unnecessary stress and embarrassment later. Besides, most people can see right through it from the get-go. So begin right this very moment by starting off all of your new friendships and relationships from this moment forward being totally honest and true to yourself and to others right out of the gate. Commit to yourself, that from now on, this is who you are and how you are going to be...Honest and Truthful!

I honestly think it is an unwritten rule that almost everybody has the ability to see through fakeness in other people. It is almost like a human intuition that comes naturally. Well since we now know that almost everyone has this ability, why continue going around being putting up a fake front? Besides having the ability to see through the fakeness, most people will not admit to you that they can see through it and will try to find a way to avoid being around you unless they need you for some reason or want you to serve one of their purposes.

A perfect example would be when I first met my (now) wife Rose through the internet, we were just chatting and talking on the phone and exchanging pictures. So I made a commitment that no matter how this new relationship I just got involved in ends up, I was going to be totally honest and down to earth. My philosophy was that I Rose to accept me for who I honestly and truly was not someone I was pretending to be because I knew in my heart that eventually she would find out the truth about me, it was just a matter of time and I did not want to risk losing Rose because of false pretenses.

As it turns out I definitely made the right decision. After one month of chatting online and talking over the phone, she flies over from Singapore to visit me for the very first time. You can only imagine how anxious, nervous, happy, and excited I was all at once waiting for her to get here. While experiencing these emotional thoughts, I also found myself experiencing a feeling of peace, calm, and serenity because I knew that I had been totally honest about myself, my situation, and what I was expecting and wanting out of this brand new relationship.

So here she was flying over to visit me for the very first time in person for who I really was, and if things worked out fantastic, and if not, well at least I was honest with myself and with Rose. Fortunately for both of us, we were both very honest – down – to – earth human beings that fell completely in love with each other. As it turns out, Rose had been involved in some rocky relationships with other guys who were not honest with her as was I with other women who were not very honest.

As a result, both Rose and I were at a point in our lives that we were tired of playing these fake relationship games and were ready to finally meet someone honest and sincere who was looking to be involved in a relationship and wanted to get married and start a new life together. So by the time we encountered each other, we were definitely ready mentally, emotionally, and honestly to meet each other. Long story short, Rose and I realized that our past relationship experiences had helped prepare us and make us ready for each other, in addition to the fact that we were both looking for the same thing in a relationship, and that we were honest with each other from the very beginning resulted in us wanting to marry each other and spend the rest of our lives together.

So when you first start dating with someone new, set the stage early on of who you really and truly are and if you have been honest with yourself and with others from the very beginning, there will be no surprises or disappointments. Frankly, if someone does not like you for who you really are, do you really want to be around that person anyway? Life is too short to spend it trying to impress other people according to their expectations. Set your own expectations of yourself then work and live according to them.

I have found that people who are true to themselves and have a definite purpose in life, and continually work at reaching that purpose, tend to be more confident, more focused, have better attitudes, are more genuine, more understanding, and more forgiving towards others. As a result, they tend to attract people to themselves as if, they were a magnet. Mostly because other people see the inner confidence in them and the fact that they are true to themselves and want to learn what this person is doing differently to be so confident.

In one sense, these types of people really are people magnets. They easily become people magnets because there are so few of them out there. Most people are not honest with themselves or other people because they portray themselves as someone other than who they really are. Are you one of these people? If so, make it your goal to begin today to start being your true self and understand that the only person you really have to impress is yourself. Do you honestly feel impressed with yourself when you pretend to be someone or something that you are really not? Of course not, because you know it is not who you really and truly are.

Start right now, this very moment being true to yourself and to others and you will notice your world beginning to change around you. People that only liked you for who you pretended to be will gradually stop hanging around you or they will begin to like you for who you really are. Either way, the only way you can ever have a lasting and meaningful relationship is by being truthful and honest with yourself and the other person in your relationship. Remember, first-and-foremost, be true to yourself, and do not worry about the people who only liked you for who you pretended to be. I call them your "pretend friends".

Eventually your "pretend friends" will fade away while people that you have never met before will suddenly start to pop into your life and become interested in you for who you really are now that you have made room in your life for them due to slowly losing your "pretend friends". They will want to be your friend because they can see that you really are true to yourself and that this is the type of person they want to be around and associated with. Now do be prepared, because it is difficult at first making this kind of change and you have to be very committed to it. The good news is that it is your decision to make this positive change, not someone else's decision. Besides, being fake is only temporary act that can cause a lot of unnecessary stress and depression, while being honest and true to yourself and others is uplifting and last forever.

Think about it...deep down inside, we all want to be honest with ourselves and with others. It is our human nature to be this way. And starting right here, right now, you too can begin being honest with yourself and with others and begin attracting true friends and lasting relationships. So the next time you feel down or depressed, ask yourself this question, am I really being true to myself and others? If not, chances are this could be one of the main reasons that you feel down or depressed?

The truth be known, most people are not impressed with who you say or think you are because they can see right through that. Rather, they are impressed with the real person that they see in you...the honest, innocent, humble, down-to-earth person in you. Most people can see past a fake front and they will not even admit to you that they know you are being fake. They may not come up to you and verbally say..."I can see that you are being fake", in fact most people will not say anything to you about it and will probably want to just avoid you as much as possible. The good news is, you can start being honest and true to yourself starting right now!

Chapter 15:

"Pace And Tone"

Pace And Tone – Did you know that the pace and tone of your conversations send a very clear signal to other people about who you are, what your intentions are, and if all you want to do is argue? Think about it for a moment. When you engage in a conversation or debate with someone, do you speak loud and fast or do you speak soft and slow? Did you know that by controlling your pace and tone, you can either prevent or defuse an argument almost instantaneously? Conversely, did you know that if you allow your pace and tone get fast and loud, you can actually provoke an argument or even a fight?

Did you also know that by speaking soft and slow, you can ultimately get more of what you are going after from another person? This is true because they feel that you are not being defensive or a threat to them, rather you portray yourself to them as being a person that controls your temper and anger. People naturally want to help other people that they perceive as being reasonable, understanding, and honest long before they will want to help someone who is causing trouble or is loud and obnoxious.

When my wife Rose and I have discussions or debates about anything, I remind her to please speak softly and slowly to prevent us from getting into a heated argument. I noticed as long as we continue talking in a soft and slow tone, we come to an agreement and find resolution fairly quickly and we are both happy. I also noticed that when our tone gets loud and our pace of speaking speeds up, we start getting louder and louder and faster and faster and the next thing you know, we are mad and yelling at each other. At this point, nothing gets resolved and we are both upset at each other for at least a couple of hours.

You see, our human nature is designed in such a way that we do not want to just give in or admit that we are wrong. This is why when we begin speaking faster and louder at someone, they feel like we are out to prove them wrong or accuse them of something, and naturally in defense, they are going to speak back at us in a faster and louder manner. Which then makes us feel like we are being accused of doing something wrong so we get even faster and louder and the cycle continues until the discussion becomes a heated argument that spins out of control.

Knowing this, you can now begin to recognize when your conversations are starting to become heated arguments, and now have the ability to take control of the entire situation simply by slowing down your pace and lowering your tone of talking. Amazingly, this starts to immediately calm the other person down and in return they will begin to slowing down their pace and lowering their tone of talking. You want to be sure to continue slowing down your pace and lowering your tones until both of you reach a reasonable pace and tone of communicating with each other again. As soon as you are certain that both of you have calmed down, you should take the initiative and let them know that you are looking for peaceful resolution, and ask them if they have any good suggestions or ideas on how both of you can resolve this matter?

If they make an unreasonable suggestion, remember to keep your pace slow and your tone low and politely ask them..."could we make it fair for both of us by doing it this way........?" As long as your pace is slow and your tone is low, they should agree with you as long as it is fair and reasonable for both of you. If they disagree and begin talking fast and loud again, let them finish speaking and then take control again by slowing down your pace and lowering your tone. The goal is to keep the conversation at a level that both of you can speak to each other peacefully without feeling intimidated or threatened. Keep slowing the pace and lowering the tone and the adrenaline levels will remain low. Somebody has got to initiate this in order for a peaceful resolution to come about, why not be the better person and let it begin with you?

So the next time you find yourself in a conversation or discussion with your boss, a family member, a friend or your fist date, remember that controlling your pace and tone controls both the momentum level of the conversation and influences the other persons pace and tone and in return, and allows you to find a more peaceful resolution faster.

Chapter 16:

"Initiating"

Initiating – Initiating is simply making the effort to do or suggest doing something. In relationships, initiating should be shared by both parties and is very important for several reasons. One, it helps the other person understand what activities you like and enjoy doing. Two, it gives direction in the relationship especially when you are just starting out in a new relationship. Three, it shares the responsibility for deciding what you are going to do. Four, it serves as a way to create a pleasant surprise for your partner when you initiate wanting to take them somewhere or do something unique or different for them. The key here is to share in the responsibility and have fun initiating activities.

This includes, going to the park, walking the dogs, working out together, dancing, going to the movies, sex, etc. The healthiest relationships consist of two individuals that share in initiating activities that both individuals enjoy doing. If one person in the relationship has to be the one to always initiate activities all of the time and the other person never initiates any of the activities, these activities start to get old and lose their appeal for the person that is always initiating the activities.

Not to mention, if after awhile, the non-initiating person continues saying no every time to the initiating person, the initiating person will eventually stop asking the non-initiating person to join them in doing these activities together. At this point, frustration can begin to build-up inside of the initiating person due to continuous feelings of rejection. Many other problems can begin to cause your relationship to lose momentum and excitement. For example, you have heard of the old saying..."do not open Pandora's box", right? Well with so many different possibilities of things that could go wrong in your relationship, allowing yourself or your partner to get to this point is like opening up Pandora's box. Who knows what could happen next.

I had experienced this type of situation firsthand with my current wife. I am always the one initiating to go to the park, go for a walk, play tennis, or drive to the mountains. On top of being the only one initiating these activities, most of the time she tells me she is not interested or not right now. It has gotten to the point that I have stopped asking her to go with me and do things together because I do not want to feel rejected by her anymore. As a result, I have built-up frustration and feel that our relationship has lost momentum and interest.

Another example of opening Pandora's box, sometimes I feel so frustrated inside because of my wife's continuous rejection, that I find myself saying things a certain way or doing things a certain way to purposely upset her. In her mind, she thinks of me as just being an inconsiderate person, when actually, that is the furthest from the truth. What she needs to do is ask herself..."is there an underlying reason that is causing him to be this way?" She would soon learn that our lack of communicating and her lack of initiating activities are the underlying problems between us. Fortunately, we decided to seek marital counseling to help identify and clarify some of these problems we were having which allowed us to correct them and now we enjoy our time with each other and know how to keep the relationship vibrant.

So do yourself and your partner a favor and be sure to take turns initiating activities that you can both do together and then make an extra effort to be sure and do them together. Even if you may not be interested in doing the activity with your partner, simply stop whatever you are doing and act as if you are interested and do the activity anyway. What you will soon discover by doing this is that you will end up having a great time doing activities together with your partner and more importantly your bond with each other will grow stronger and stronger with every activity and your relationship will prosper.

Chapter 17:

"Human Nature"

Human Nature – Most people believe that human nature is hard to predict and in some cases this may be true. For the most part though, all humans have basic needs that have to be met and as a result can be predictable. The basic human needs in life include, air, food, water, shelter, love, and money. Love is our focus here for this discussion. Along with the basic need for love, come the emotions and desires for love, and the fulfillment of love.

Human nature can sometimes be very irrational, meaning that some people will do just about anything to fulfill their basic need for love. This is extremely important to understand, because if the person you are married to or involved with cannot fulfill your emotional cravings, needs, and wants for love, human nature will take over and you will eventually begin seeking out someone else that can fulfill your emotional cravings for love. Conversely, if you cannot fulfill your partners needs, desires, and wants for love, they will also begin seeking out someone else that can fulfill their emotional cravings for love.

If your relationship gets to this point or has already gotten to this point, chances are very good that you will either need to seek professional counseling or have some major changes take place to keep your relationship from spiraling downward and out of control. In my case, I began drinking to cover up my frustration. I started drinking so much that my wife decided she was leaving me and not coming back until I quit drinking. Believe it or not, I had so much frustration built-up inside of me that I actually felt relieved with her being gone for two days and did not have the urge to drink.

The more I thought about it, the more I realized that my urge to drink excessively stemmed directly from the frustration I was experiencing inside and that the frustration I felt inside came from the feeling that my emotional cravings for love were not being met. I then realized that the main reason my emotional cravings for love were not being met is because I was the only one in our relationship that was initiating activities and I was constantly being rejected by my wife whenever I would initiate these activities. This is a classic example of problems being caused by "underlying reasons" which you will learn more about in a later section. My human nature had kicked in and was looking for a way to suppress my feelings of hurt and rejection and for me alcohol seemed to be the best vehicle to accomplish this.

The secret to human nature is an open-minded open line of communication, initiation, and honesty. Simply by asking your partner..."sweetheart, is there anything that I can do for you that would allow me to please you more, either emotionally or sexually?" If they say no, look them straight in the eyes and softly ask them... "are you sure there is nothing else I can do to please you more?" If they still say no, ask them..."if at any point you find that there is something that I could do to please you more, would you please come share it with me?"

Several very important things are going to happen when you do this. One, your partner is going to feel elated that you were concerned enough to ask about better pleasing them. Two, you left the door open for them to come back to you at a later time and let you know what it is they really want you to do for them since they may have been a little embarrassed at first. Three, you set the stage for your partner to become more interested in making sure that all of your pleasures are also being met.

Have fun with it, take turns pleasing each other, one night it is your turn to please your partner, the next night it is their turn to please you. Whatever it is that turns them on, be open-minded and respect them for it. Everybody has something special that they would like to have done to them or for them that they find pleasing. Anyone that says "no", is either too embarrassed to say yes or has not discovered their ultimate pleasure yet. If this is the case, you can help them experiment and discover their ultimate pleasure. So remember to be sure and keep your partner's emotional cravings for love satisfied and that way you will not have to worry about them wanting to be with someone else that can.

Chapter 18:

"Seeds"

Seeds – We all know that seeds are something that you put into the ground and then plants begin growing, right? Well did you know that we can actually plant seeds of thought in someone's mind and that things begin gradually changing or happening the moment we plant these seeds of thought? The difference here is that the type of seeds we are capable of planting in someone's mind, consist of "thoughts". So, for right now, we are going to talk about the seeds that you plant in someone's mind or "seeds of thought".

Thoughts are a type of seed that one person can plant into the mind of another. Unlike normal crop seeds, these seeds of thought that can be planted into someone else's mind can vary on how long it takes for these seeds to mature depending on what type of seed you planted and the type of person. For example, let us say that you really want to marry someone and yet you know that they are not quite ready for the commitment. You could start to plant the seed of thought in their mind by saying..."you know I have never been this happy being involved in a relationship as I am with you. If you ever decided to get married, it sure would make me the happiest person on earth if you decided to pick me to be your soul mate".

In effect, what you are doing here is subconsciously telling this person that you would love to be married to them without applying unbearable pressure on them. Now you might think it went in one ear and out the other, but actually it got stored and processed in their subconscious memory. All you have to do is continue being yourself, and make sure that the relationship remains interesting and pleasurable for both of you.

This does not mean that you have to start having sex if you have not previously engaged in sex with this person. It simply means that as long as the relationship between both of you remains interesting, vibrant and fun to be in, this person will one day realize that if they do not commit to you and marry you, then someone else will, and chances are they do not want to lose you to someone else. Especially if you are vibrant and fun to be with...so when the time is right, plant your seeds and let nature take its course. All you need to do is keep the relationship entertaining and fun.

So the next time you get involved in a relationship and feel that you cannot live without this person and want to marry them, remember to properly plant your seeds of thought without applying pressure, then be patient, keep the relationship interesting, and let nature take her course.

Chapter 19:

"Patience & Faith"

Patience & Faith – Patience and faith go hand in hand with planting seeds. Once you have sewn your seeds in your partner's mind, you have to be patient and have faith that your partner will become conscious and aware of the seeds that you planted in their mind and will eventually act upon them. If for marriage, may the good Lord be willing and allow you both to grow old together and play with your grandchildren. So often I meet and see people that want things in life and after a few short exchanges of words, it is very clear that these people lack faith in the belief of that which they claim to want so badly.

Truly nothing of great value comes easily. This includes a meaningful or long-lasting marriage or relationship. You may have heard of the old saying..."lucky is the man who has good wife". Well what they do not tell you is that the man and wife went through a lot of trials and tribulations in their life together that probably still continue to this day. What they also do not tell you is that it took a lot of patience from each of them to learn to get through their problems and probably just as much faith to visualize seeing themselves in the future where they had gotten past most of their problems.

Most people make the mistake in relationships of thinking that just because they want their partner to give up a certain habit or action that they perceive to be negative in their partner, that their partner should start acting upon their wish immediately to get rid of their bad habit or action, and as a result, they expect sudden change. When this does not happen according to the expecting partner's time-frame, they will usually get impatient and begin growing angry towards the offending partner. What the expecting partner fails to recognize is that they are dealing with human nature and just like that certain habit was formed over a period of time, it will also take a period of time for their partner to break that certain habit.

Rather than being upset and frustrated at the offending partner for not immediately breaking their perceived bad habit, you should be patient and supportive and have faith that the habit will be broken. I have learned this first-hand with my wife because she has an approach that is completely ineffective. She'll want to yell and scream at me, thinking that she could scare me out of doing something. Here again, she fails to recognize that she is dealing with various levels of human nature. Meaning that when she yells and screams at me, it has just the opposite effect of what her intentions are. Rather than listening attentively, my mind and level of interest in what she is saying begin to close down and as a result I fail to process what she is saying.

A good example of what would be a much more effective approach for her to take with me would be to calmly say to me..."honey, there is something that is really been bothering me. I have noticed that you do not take the trash out every Friday like you used to. I was wondering if you would please remember to make sure to take the trash out every Friday to keep the house from smelling up?" Now this approach would have a far more reaching impact on making sure that I get back into the habit of taking out the trash than any amount of yelling or screaming she projects towards me.

This approach may need to be repeated several or more times in the same calm manner to help someone completely break a habit that you find offensive. You can use this approach to help someone stop drinking too much, stop smoking so much, helping out around the house, cutting the grass, stop flirting with other people, stop cussing, etc. etc. The key here is to always remain extremely calm while explaining how you feel and remember that it takes patience and faith.

The reason this approach is much more effective than yelling or screaming at someone is because instead of trying and failing to pound your anger into someone else's mind about how you feel, you are subconsciously and calmly putting the offending person in the position of seeing and feeling what you see and feel from their own perspective and by so doing, you are allowing them to realize by themselves that something needs to be done to correct this problem. Instead of experiencing a feeling of being ridiculed, you allow them to experience a feeling of awareness.

So please learn to recognize that when yelling, screaming, and getting upset fails to help someone break an undesired habit. Use this more effective approach by applying patience and faith along with a calm explanation of what's bothering you and why it is bothering you. Remember, it will not happen over night so remain calm, be patient, and have faith because most habit take an average of 30 days to form or break. Eventually, all of their really bad habits can be corrected. At the same time, you want to be careful about asking your partner to make too many changes because otherwise they will not be the person you met and fell in love with.

Chapter 20:

"Because"

Because – The word "Because" is an effective transition to use in your conversations because it allows you to explain to someone the reason or purpose behind something. For example, if I asked you..."can you pick me up tomorrow at 3:00PM?" You may or may not be very inclined to pick me up. However, if I asked you..."can you pick me up tomorrow at 3:00PM because my car will be in the shop and I need a ride home?" Chances are you will be a lot more inclined to pick me up tomorrow at 3:00PM because you now know the reason or purpose behind me needing a ride.

Another example of how the word "because" can make your conversations more effective is by using it after you make a statement or claim. For example if I wanted to explain to you how good my product or service was, I basically have two ways of doing it. One, "we offer the best customer service and pricing in town." Or, Two, "we offer the best customer service and pricing in town "because" we buy direct from the wholesaler and stand 100% behind every product we sell." Obviously, number two puts you a lot more at ease and makes you feel more comfortable in dealing with me "because" I went a little bit further in explaining the reason or purpose behind my customer service.

The same rule applies to everything that you talk about to everybody. For example: Let us pretend for a moment that you are in a situation whereby the person you are interested in is also interested in dating someone else and is having a difficult time contemplating who to date. Knowing this, you have an opportunity to persuade the person you are interested in to decide to date you as opposed to the other person. In this situation, what would you say and how would you say it? Remember, you only have one shot at convincing this person to date just you. I will list two examples of what to say and how to say it and you decide which is the most effective in convincing the person you are interested in.

Example one: "I know that you are facing a really tough decision in trying to decide who you want to date and have a relationship with. I think I can save you some time and frustration by letting you know that I would by far be the best person for you to date and have a relationship with."

Example two: "I know that you are facing a really tough decision in trying to decide who you want to date and have a relationship with. I think I can save you some time and frustration by letting you know that I would by far be the best person for you to date and have a relationship with "because" I have been through the ropes before and I know for a fact that you are exactly the person that I have been looking for all along. Besides, I know how to treat a lady / man and if you are ever feeling down, I will always be there to pick you up." "Can we make a commitment together to just date each other over the next 30 days to prove that we were meant to be together?" (small commitments leading up to larger commitments)

You can begin to see how important the word "because" can become in your conversations, right? So remember, whenever you are about to make a statement or claim, always follow-up your claim or statement with the word "because" and let the person know the reason or purpose behind your statement or claim.

Chapter 21:

"Which Means To You"

Which Means To You – Which means to you is one of the most effective transitions in communicating that can be used to keep someone's interest in what you are talking about. Think about it for a moment! When you spend your time telling someone about something that you have done or experienced, after a while they are probably thinking in the back of their mind..."so what" or "who cares" or "like I really care what you experienced", what they are really thinking or wanting to say is..."what does that do for me or what does that mean to me?"

Again, we are dealing with human nature and most people are going to have the same reaction. You have seen it before, where someone is bragging about their accomplishments, or achievements, or paycheck etc., while the people listening are thinking who really cares? Or what does that do for me? So when you find yourself involved in your next conversation bragging about yourself or tooting your own horn, keep this in mind that everyone is tuned in to their very own radio station..."WIIFM". Which stands for "What's In It For Me"?

One way you can help prevent other people from feeling this way as well as keep them interested in what you are saying, is to use the transition "which means to you". For example, "John, I caught the biggest fish in the lake yesterday using just my Spincaster and an eight pound fishing line." Well at this point John is probably thinking..."who cares". So a more effective way to share my story and keep John interested is by saying..."John, I caught the biggest fish in the lake yesterday using just my spincaster and an eight pound fishing line, which means that the next time you go fishing there John, you should use the eight pound fishing line instead of the ten pound fishing line Spincaster and you will be able to catch some of the biggest fish in the lake as well.

Now you can clearly see that John was more interested in what I have to say because I have included something in my story that was for John's benefit. This is an effective way to keep your conversations interesting whether you are speaking to your friends, spouse, family, or a new date. Do not just tell your story, tell your story and how it applies or what it means to the person to talking to. You will start to find that more people are interested in your conversations and what you have to say.

So remember, the next time you want to brag about yourself, or toot your own horn in front of other people, do it in such a way so that you do not come across as someone bragging in front of other people. More importantly, find a way to include a benefit in your conversation for the people you are talking to and you will find that they are a lot more interested in what you have to say.

Chapter 22:

"The Benefit To You"

The Benefit To You – "The Benefit To You" is another effective transition that can be used in your conversations with other people. Remember, everyone is tuned into their own radio station "WIIFM" (What's In It For Me). This means that everyone is constantly looking for the benefit for themselves in just about everything they participate in. This could be a job, a date, a marriage, a vacation, a conversation, you name it. If you can make it easy for the people you are talking to, to see the benefit in what you are talking about, you have 90% of the battle won.

For example, let us pretend that you are in a situation whereby you just met someone very attractive both physically and mentally. In fact they are so attractive that you just cannot stop thinking about them and you want to make sure they stay interested in you long enough to realize how strongly your feelings are for them. Knowing that once they realize how attracted you are to them, they will be just as attracted to you. What would you say to this extremely attractive person and how would you say it? Remember, you are going to be experiencing feelings of nervousness, excitement, joy, and scared all in one.

So here is an example of what to say and how to say it. "Please forgive me for being so nervous in front of you. I cannot help but feel so nervous because I just met the most attractive person on earth and I feel completely speechless. The reason that I am sharing this with you is because that most attractive person on earth happens to be you and I cannot think of any fancy lines to tell you to try to sweep you off of your feet. In fact the only thing I think of right now, is being extremely honest with you. I guess you could say that the "benefit" to you is that whenever I feel this nervous, scared, and excited all a the same time about something, it is impossible for me to do anything else besides tell the truth and be honest."

"Now that I have completely made a fool of myself in front you from being so nervous and scared, would it be possible for me to meet up with you later for some coffee or tea and get to know you a little better?" Now one of several things is going to happen at this point. One, the person you are attracted to is going to be completely understanding about you being nervous and will probably feel flattered and will agree to meet you for coffee or tea later. Or, Two, they may not be interested in you at all and not agree to meet you for coffee or tea. The fact of the matter is that you will never know unless you make the attempt to introduce yourself to this person both properly and politely.

The reason I know this approach does work is because I personally experienced it. Except I was with a friend of mine at a bar having a few drinks after work. As I began walking towards the men's bathroom, coming out of the women's bathroom walks one of the most beautiful Asian-American women I have ever seen on this planet. I immediately experienced feelings of excitement, joy, nervousness and scared all at the same time. The feelings were so intense and overbearing that I felt like someone had just hit me in the chest and knocked me back about ten feet just from being in her presence. I literally had trouble breathing from being so nervous just from seeing her walk towards me.

I came out of the bathroom and immediately went over to my friend to explain to him what had just happened to me and how nervous I was over the thought of introducing myself to her. In fact I was so nervous, I could not turn around to look at her while she was looking in my direction. Finally after about 20 minutes of experiencing these awkward feelings, my friend pushed me over towards her where she had three other guys around her talking to her in the middle of the bar. After I had bumped into her from being pushed by my friend, she turned around and looked at me as if I had just disturbed her.

I immediately apologized and said to her "I could not keep from noticing how absolutely beautiful you are and how extremely nervous I am right now in front of you. I don't have some fancy lines to tell you like I want to show you the stars or anything like that. I was just wondering if I could have the opportunity to meet up with you for either coffee or tea and get to know you better?" Amazingly, she said, "that would be fine". I felt like I just conquered the world. The next day, I called her and invited her out to dinner and once she saw how attracted I was to her, she began having mutual feelings of attraction towards me and we dated each other for almost eight months until we realized there were some major differences between our lifestyles.

She knew by the way that I presented myself, and what I had said to her, that I was being honest and that the benefit to her was that she was going to be with someone that was going to be honest and truthful with her. So remember, the next time you are in a situation like this, be honest and let the other person see what the benefit is to them. You never know what someone else is going to say or think about wanting to date you or be with you. You can however control what you say and how you say it to help increase your chances of getting exactly what you are focused on going after.

Chapter 23:

"What You Are Speaks So Loudly"

What You Are Speaks So Loudly – This is another extremely important lesson for you to understand. The complete phrase is "what you are speaks so loudly that I cannot hear what you are saying." In effect, what this means is that no matter how often or how loudly you "try" to explain who you are or who you think you are to other people, people are actually ignoring your words because they can see with their own eyes "who" you really are. Therefore, they do not even listen to your words because they can see who you really are through your actions. Basically, it means..."your actions speak louder than your words".

This can be positive or negative and especially happens a lot to people who are always bragging about themselves, people that act as if they know-it-all, people that have bad tempers, people that are selfish and people that greedy to name a few on the negative side. While at the same time, it happens to people who are genuinely nice, concerned for others, have compassion, use actions instead of words, go out of their way to help other people to name a few on the positive side. So be very careful to make sure that you are a person whose actions are positive and do not let yourself fall into the negative category.

Have you ever noticed someone who does something nice and then they turn around and make a big deal about it because they want everyone else know about it? Then on the other hand, you have people who repeatedly do nice things and never say a word about it. Can you see the difference here? It is better to be the person who does something nice and does not say a word to anyone else about it because eventually, people will start to notice what type of person you really are through your actions. Once they know, they will be sure to tell other people and soon the word gets around what type of person your really, whether good or bad.

Now this does not mean that you have to go out of your way just to help people out for the sake of trying to gain a good reputation. It just simply means that when the opportunity arises and you have the ability to help out, quietly lend a hand along with a smile and help the other person out. Not only does the person you are helping appreciate the help, you will feel great about yourself for being able to help them. Besides, the Universe usually gives back to us more than we give out whether good or bad, and you never know, you might be the person that needs the help one day. Did you help out others when you had your chance? If so, chances are good that help will be readily available for you when you most need it.

So remember, the next time you find yourself in a situation where someone needs your help and you have the ability to help that person out, quietly lend your hand along with a smile. Above all, do not make a big deal about helping the person out and do not expect anything in return from the person. You will gain a reputation of someone that is helpful, kind, and generous without having to say a word to anyone else. You will also have help readily available to you whenever you need it and you will be more attractive as a human being.

Chapter 24:

Do You Think or Do You Feel? – Well, do you think or feel? What is the difference? It sounds like a silly question right? Let me explain to you why it is so important. Let us suppose for a moment that you were going out on your first date with someone that you really find attractive and while at dinner, you begin to engage in conversation with the intent of starting to get small commitments and to find out more about this person. If any of your questions involves their opinion, you had better know the right way to ask them for it. The reason this is so important is because some people actually become offensive when you ask them to give their opinion especially when it relates to a touchy subject such as politics, religion, government, world issues etc if you do not ask for it in the proper way. This often happens because some people feel like they are being put in the spotlight and are expected to give a "right or wrong" answer.

So depending on the way that you ask the question will depend on the type of answer you get back and whether you made someone feel uncomfortable or not. For example, if you asked your new dating partner at dinner the following question..."so what do you "think" about the new government that the United States is helping to build in Iraq since Saddam Hussein is now gone?" Do not be surprised if you may get an answer mixed with negative feelings and emotions not to mention make the person feel uncomfortable. A more appropriate way to ask the question for example would be like..."so tell me, "in your opinion", how do you "feel" about the new government that the United States is helping to build in Iraq?"

Can you begin to feel and see the difference here? When you start off a question by asking someone…"what do you think?", most people will immediately begin to feel like there has got to be a right or wrong answer. However, if you ask someone…"how do you feel about, or in your opinion, how do you feel about?" you put the person at ease because you are only asking them for their opinion and not a perceived right or wrong answer. Almost everyone is willing to give you their opinion pertaining to specific topic or subject long before they are willing to tell you what they think about it.

Additionally, It is a much smoother way to help the other person open up and share their feelings with you, which is ultimately what you are after, right? So remember, the next time you find yourself in conversation, be sure to ask the other person either…"how do you feel about….or, in your opinion, how do you feel about?" and you will notice two important things will happen. One, you will keep the other person from feeling like they are being put on the spotlight, which feels very uncomfortable. Two, you will help the other person open up much quicker and share their true feelings with you and find you more attractive as a result.

Chapter 25:

"Act As If"

Act As If – That is right! Act as if. Act as if everything is going to end up wonderfully on your first date even if it is pouring down rain, or the restaurant is completely packed and cannot accommodate your reservation, or you get a flat tire on the way to the restaurant with your new date in the car. Act as if everything is going to end up wonderfully. You do this for several very good reasons.

One, people admire someone who can keep their cool in heated situations. Two, things just happen in life, so learn to accept it. Three, it conveys a feeling of confidence to your new date. Four, it keeps them calm and relaxed. Five, it shows them that you can think quickly on your feet. Six, your example will inspire them to be the same way if they are ever in such a situation. Seven, your ability to handle the situation well might be all it takes for them to take a serious liking to you and want to continue dating you.

Regardless of what the circumstances are, keep your cool and act as if everything is going to end up ok. Because ultimately it really will. Temporary setbacks are just that, a temporary setback. It is not the end! Relax, make the most of the situation and act as if everything is going to turn out just fine. To your amazement, the moment you begin to "act as if" and accept it as being true, you will almost immediately notice that everything really will turn out just fine and that a bad situation begins turning for the better the very moment you realize it, accept it, and believe it to be true. Also remember to have patience and faith in yourself and in your abilities and if it helps you, use your mind to visualize what you want the end result to be.

So remember, the next time you are encountered with a bad situation, accept it, and immediately begin to deal with it while remaining calm and "Act As If" everything is going to turn out just fine.

Chapter 26:

"CHOICES"

CHOICES – We all have the ability to make our own CHOICES in life. For some reason most of the people that I have met so far seem to believe that things just happen to them in life without any rhyme or reason. Standing from the outside looking in, it is easy to understand why some people would feel this way. Taking a closer look however reveals some startling information that most people would have trouble accepting.

For example, most people look at someone who's rich or famous and immediately think to themselves..."that person sure is lucky, I'd love to live their life or be that person." While this is great for fantasizing, one also needs to realize that this rich or famous person is exactly where they are because they have made certain CHOICES throughout their life to live their life a certain way and to continually sacrifice and do things a certain way until they became famous or rich. These people make a conscious decision where they want to go in life and every single day that they wake up, they CHOOSE to keep doing the things that count the most and that will ultimately keep bringing their goal closer and closer, day by day.

Please understand that all of us have CHOICES to make every single day of our lives. In fact, did you realize that even if you CHOOSE not to decide on something, you still have made a CHOICE? Therefore, it would be better to decide on the best possible CHOICE that you can make than leave things to chance? So often I hear people saying or commenting..."I am not going to CHOOSE which side I want to be on, or I will let Mother Nature or God CHOOSE for me." What they do not realize is that by deciding not to CHOOSE, they are still making a CHOICE. Whether you CHOOSE to make a decision or not, a CHOICE is still being made.

Since a choice is going to be made either way, it only makes sense to choose the option that is in your best interest? This especially applies to your choice of words or attitudes. For example, I have to keep reminding my wife that she should choose to control her temper and the words that she uses a little better. For some reason, she does not feel that she is in control of her temper, words, and attitude. I keep asking her..."if you are not in charge of them then who is?" Like most people, she has not quite learned or accepted that she is in total control of her actions, attitudes, words, feelings, or temper. By failing to choose to control her attitude, she is actually making a choice to have a bad attitude, or temper, or words.

The key here is to always remember that you are totally in control of your thoughts, feelings, actions, and attitudes and that you can actually control the outcome or the end result of a situation depending on the choices you make. A lot of people are scared to accept this fact because they do not want to accept the responsibility that comes along with it. It is much easier to sit back and say..."the reason I said this or did that is because of what you said or did to me." That is simply failing to accept responsibility for your own words and actions and trying to shift the blame on someone else because you failed to choose a better outcome or end result.

So the next time you engage in conversation with someone you really like or are interested in, make sure that you CHOOSE your attitudes, words, actions, and emotions very carefully because it could mean the difference between winning or losing a second date, a contest, a job promotion, a sale, a contract etc.. At the same time, notice how well the people you engage in conversations with, choose their words, attitudes, actions, and emotions, and see if they accept full responsibility then ask yourself..."do they know and understand what I now know and understand about the importance of accepting responsibility for my choices? Or that each individual is in complete control of their own choices?" Most people do not realize this or do not want to accept the responsibility for it.

So I leave you with one final question in this section about "Choices"... "If you are not in charge of your choices, then who is?"

Chapter 27:

LUCK – Everyone has used the word LUCK or LUCKY at some point or time throughout their life, right? The problem with the use and understanding of the word LUCK is that most people do not know what LUCK really stands for nor do they understand what the true meaning is. As a result, the word LUCK gets misused repeatedly and is completely misunderstood. Unless you know the true meaning of the word LUCK, forget whatever you have learned about it and let us start all over.

What LUCK really means is Laboring Under Correct Knowledge. LUCK is what happens to someone who has totally prepared themselves for an opportunity and the opportunity arises. Hence, LUCK is when preparation meets opportunity and opportunity is abundant and all around us all the time. The real question is..."are you prepared for the opportunity?" Take dating for example, did you take time to learn how present yourself, how to conduct yourself, how to have a meaningful conversation, how to dress, and how to impress? If so, then other people will say that you are LUCKY when you end meeting and dating the person of your dreams.

If on the other hand, you did not prepare yourself to take advantage of the opportunity, then chances are things will not turn out so well and you will feel UNLUCKY. You see, here again you are in control and can choose to prepare yourself for the opportunity of an exciting date and the end result will be determined by how well your prepared yourself. In addition to dating, this also holds true for obtaining a job, promotions, graduating, buying, selling, negotiating etc. Practically every advancement or opportunity you take advantage of in life will mostly be determined by how well you prepared yourself for the opportunity.

So do you feel LUCKY? It is not hard to tell if you are prepared for an opportunity. It comes from an inner feeling that you get after spending time preparing yourself for an opportunity. Either you either feel really confident about an opportunity, and have a "yes I am ready" attitude or you will feel like "I will give it my best shot and see what happens" type of attitude. Whatever the end result is, accept full responsibility and either embrace the opportunity because you prepared for it or go back to the drawing board and better prepare yourself for the next time. Whatever happens, keep a positive and cheerful attitude and remember that you will have many other opportunities to prepare for if this one did not turn out the way you wanted.

So the next time you hear someone say "he or she sure is LUCKY". You will know better and realize what LUCK really means and more importantly, what it really takes to be considered LUCKY. Most importantly, remember, Good Luck or Bad Luck...there is no such thing. People will use these terms to try and psyche you out mentally. Remember, you are in full control of your thoughts, emotions, actions, and attitudes. So choose to disregard being psyched out by someone else who is less informed about what LUCK really means and ask this one question. How well did you prepare yourself for the opportunity before you? Now this is how you take full responsibility for your actions rather than buying into some psyched-out fairytale belief.

Chapter 28:

"Attitude"

Attitude – Everyone has one of these...an attitude that is. Some of us have a pleasant attitude, some of us have a mean attitude, and some of us do not even know that we have an attitude. You may have heard of the saying that "attitude determines altitude"? Well it is absolutely true! You can sort of look at it like this. Bad attitude equals bad results, fair or average attitude equals fair or average results, good attitude equals good results, and great attitude equals great results. Life does not play any favorites when it comes to people. Therefore your results will be in direct proportion to your attitude.

Life is like a merciless mirror. Whatever we are at this moment or have chosen to become is reflected right directly back at us. One way to quickly test your attitude is ask yourself..."do people smile when they see me coming?" If so, chances are you have a good attitude, if not, chances are you have a bad attitude. Regardless of what your current attitude is, you can begin to improve your attitude starting right now. The most important step towards improving your attitude is to begin at this very moment to accept complete and full responsibility for all of your thoughts, actions, emotions, and words. The key here is to realize and accept that you are in total control and responsible for all of your thoughts, actions, emotions, and words. This is a fact!

Once you accept this responsibility, the next step is to begin choosing how you want to handle this responsibility. Meaning, do you want to use it to treat people nicely or badly? Just as important, how do you want to feel about yourself, positively or negatively? Since you are now in full control of your thoughts, actions, words, and emotions, you can now choose and decide how you want to think, feel, act, speak and conduct yourself. It is almost like you are your own movie producer or music conductor. What type of person do you want to be in your own movie or what type of music do you want to play... sad, happy, or enthusiastic? Whatever your choice is, that is exactly what other people will see in you.

If for any reason, you find it difficult at first to get started in a new and better direction with your new and better attitude, remember to always "act as if". Act as if you are already in possession of that new great attitude. What you will discover by acting as if, is that you will begin to become the person that you envision with a new and great attitude and as time passes, you will soon realize that you are that person with the great attitude. So begin choosing right now to have a new and great attitude and act as if you are already in possession of it and soon it will be yours.

If you are concerned about what your past friendships or relationships will think or feel about you suddenly wanting to make a change, forget about them! If they liked who you were before, will not they like you even more with a better and more positive attitude? If not, chances are they are only trying to keep you down or hold you back and that is not healthy. I would much rather be around a group of people that are positive and have great attitudes than tolerate people that are always negative and have poor attitudes. The choice is yours to make and keep.

Now that you have decided to improve your attitude and take it to the next level, the next step is to realize that similar to being involved in a relationship, it takes ongoing daily effort. Did you realize that how you think or feel the first five to ten minutes after waking up in the morning sets the stage for your attitude for the rest of the day? Now that you know this, you can now choose to begin to take specific action to make sure that you start off the day with a great attitude that continues all day long.

The best way to accomplish this is to start off every day with a positive or motivating self-induced thought or saying. Personally, I start off the first waking moments of every day with a couple of mantras. They include: "What a glorious day filled with love, opportunity, happiness, and success", "I love myself and many great miracles are now happening", "I am grateful and I expect to succeed". This sets the stage for my entire day and regardless of whether the sun is shining or if it is pouring down rain, I have an outstanding day full of optimism, gratitude, and cheerfulness. Needless to say, I am smiling all day long as a result and a lot of people call me smiley.

Some of the hidden benefits that you will gain by living this way include. One, you are genuinely a much happier person and people notice it immediately. Two, your stress levels will begin to decrease almost immediately. Three, people will be more attracted to you. Four, you will find yourself smiling a lot more and other people smiling back at you. Five, you will notice that you start to get more of what you want out of life faster. Six, you will become an inspiration to the people around you to improve their attitudes. Seven, you will no longer be bothered by petty little circumstances. Eight, you will be more forgiving and understanding towards others. Nine, you will go out on more dates. Ten, you will get hired and promoted faster.

This is not to say that you still will not have occasional bad days. There will just be a lot less of them. Also this does not mean that you should go around proving that you are a positive and optimistic person with a great attitude and trying to get everyone else to be the same way. All you really have to do, is quietly make your own improvements and adjustments and everyone else will start to notice without you saying a word to them. Then, what you have become will be speaking so loudly, that you will not have to tell other people what you are, they will see it in you. So be sure to start off each morning in the right direction by choosing to control and direct your thoughts, actions, and emotions in a positive direction and watch the world around you begin to change right before your very own eyes.

Chapter 29:

"Enthusiasm"

Enthusiasm – One of the fastest ways to get yourself out of a rut or a lull is with the use of enthusiasm. Enthusiasm is simply digging deep down inside of yourself and generating a feeling of complete excitement about the opportunities surrounding you. Remember, there are always opportunities surrounding you! All you have to do is take notice of them and be prepared for them. Enthusiasm is also contagious and makes other people enjoy being around you. Not to mention, other people quickly notice someone who is full of enthusiasm as soon as they see them. It is almost as if you were wearing a big sign on your forehead that says "I am excited about life" and almost immediately other people are attracted to you like a magnet!

It is easy to spot someone full of enthusiasm because they will be bubbling over with excitement and joy about an opportunity they have either just discovered or have known about for quite awhile. Whether they have a new date, a new job, a new promotion, a new car, a new house, or a newborn baby, you will see them radiating with excitement and joy. Believe this or not, as human beings, all of us have the ability to self-induce enthusiasm within ourselves whenever we choose almost instantaneously. So feel free to use plenty of enthusiasm in your life because there is no lack of it and all of us have access to it whenever we choose. The key is in knowing how to conjure it up to make it work for you.

The secret to conjuring up enthusiasm is in understanding how our feelings and emotions work and realizing that we have control over them. Just as we have the ability to make choices regarding our thoughts, actions, words, and emotions, we also have the ability to control our enthusiasm. Enthusiasm is nothing more than an emotion that expresses extreme happiness, excitement and joy. The best way to self-induce enthusiasm is done through a three-step process.

First, think about something totally exciting and positive and just imagine that it is happening for you right now at this very moment. Second, psyche yourself up by telling your mind and imagining that you now feel full of joy, happiness and excitement right now at this very moment. Third, consciously choose to go through the motions of being enthusiastic by simply acting as if you were already full of enthusiasm. By doing this for several minutes you will suddenly begin to smile and feel enthusiasm running throughout your entire body.

Our subconscious minds do not know the difference between right and wrong or real and fake. It only knows what we tell it or program into it as being true. Therefore, the secret is in the ability to use your conscious mind to inject a thought that you find positive, exciting, and stimulating into your subconscious mind while temporarily believing that this thought is new thought is true for a period of several minutes until the thought transcends into a feeling of excitement and joy throughout your entire body at which point it becomes a real experience. Then continue visualizing and replaying this exciting experience through your conscious mind over and over again for as long as you would like to remain enthusiastic.

Please understand that because of the way we humans are made up genetically, we can only experience one type of emotion at a time. Meaning that you cannot be happy and sad both at the same time. At any given moment, you are either happy or sad or angry, and yet you cannot experience more than one of these emotions at any given time. Just like you cannot smile and feel sad or angry at the same time. The moment you begin to smile, your anger subsides. Therefore, by choosing to think of something happy and enthusiastic, you will begin to smile and feel happy inside. So the next time you are about to go out on a date or meet someone new, choose to make yourself look and feel enthusiastic by injecting positive, happy, and enthusiastic thoughts into your mind and you will make a great first impression and attract more people as if you were a magnet. Remember, how you choose to feel or let yourself feel is entirely up to you. Since the choice is yours, why not choose to be happy and enthusiastic?

Chapter 30:

"Psychosomatic"

Psychosomatic – Did you know that when you CHOOSE to allow yourself to feel sad, your face looks sad and when you CHOOSE to be happy, your face looks happy? The reason for this is because we are all psychosomatic. Psychosomatic simply means that our moods and emotions are in direct correlation with our thoughts and expressed outwardly. More importantly, these moods and emotions are carried out through our facial expressions and body language in such a way that it lets the rest of the world around us know, exactly how we are feeling. For example, have you ever noticed that when one of your friends or family members are sad, you can almost tell immediately without them saying a word to you, right? That is because their thoughts are controlling their moods and emotions, which are being carried out and expressed through their facial expressions and body language. This is why it is very important to control your thoughts, moods, and emotions, because everyone else around you can see what you are thinking simply by observing your facial expressions and body language.

Another reason why understanding what psychosomatic means is so important to you is because it also applies to sickness, diseases, enthusiasm, anxiety, frustration, hypertension, good health, atrophy, etc., meaning that if you continually think to yourself that you feel like you are going to get sick, then chances are very strong that you will end up becoming sick. On the other hand, if you control your thoughts by continually reminding yourself that your body feels healthy and strong and full of energy, then not only will you project those feelings and emotions through your facial expressions and body language, your body will actually begin to feel healthier and stronger and full of energy. Believe it or not, your thoughts are very powerful...especially when it comes to your health and survival.

Let us demonstrate this very quickly so that you will fully understand how this process works. Stand in front a mirror and think of a sour tasting lemon, what is your immediate reaction? What happened to your facial expression? Next, think of peeling and taking a big bite out of the sour tasting lemon, what is your immediate reaction then? What happened to your facial expression? Can you see that just by the mere thought alone of tasting the juices from the sour tasting lemon would make your mouth start to pucker up? Let's take a look at the facts. As you FOCUSED your thoughts to think about tasting or biting into a sour tasting lemon, your mouth and facial expressions puckered up.

This is an example of what happens when YOU FOCUS your mind and thoughts on certain things either consciously or subconsciously. For example, if I said to you, "think about smiling", chances are you will begin smiling because that is the immediate conscious thought going through your mind. Your facial expressions are in direct correlation to your thoughts, whether good or bad. Another important fact to remember is that the human mind cannot process thoughts of happiness and sadness at the same exact time and that it is a CHOICE that has to be made whether to focus on something sad or happy. This means that if you find yourself feeling sad or depressed, take action at that moment and begin to make a conscious decision to change your thoughts to something more positive and joyful and follow through with it with full FOCUS.

Remember, the next time you find yourself in a situation where you need to control your emotions or feelings or facial expressions, think of something positive and cheerful and you will notice yourself starting to feel cheerful, happy, and smiling. So on your next dating opportunity, be sure to think of happy and positive things in your life and your date will see a happy and positive person in you that they will find more interesting and attractive.

Chapter 31:

"Be Here NOW In The Present Moment"

Be Here NOW In The Present Moment – So often I find that when people who are engaged in conversations with me, are drifting off thinking about doing something else or being somewhere else. I sometimes wondered if I am a boring person to talk to or did they just learn a bad habit that has gotten out of control. I then realized that when they began doing something else or got to the other place they were thinking about while in conversation with me, they begin thinking back about the conversation they were having with me earlier in the day. What these people do not realize is that they are literally robbing themselves of the opportunity to fully enjoy each moment that they are experiencing right then and there. This happens because they fail to realize that they are in full control of their thoughts, emotions, and actions.

As a result of not controlling their attention and listening skills, they are missing many opportunities right before their very own eyes, whether they prepared themselves or not for the opportunities. For example they might be thinking of going to the park when they are at work and when they get to the park, they are thinking about working. What they should to learn to do is control their thoughts, emotions, and actions and "be here now in the present moment". That is, they need to learn to take control of their thoughts and keep themselves fully engrossed and engaged and FOCUSED in whatever activity they are supposed to be doing at that very moment in time. Otherwise, they may begin to feel guilty because they are not getting their work done when they should be working and they cannot relax while they are supposed to be resting at the park.

This can be resolved simply by bringing your conscious mind into the present moment of an activity that you are supposed to be engaged in. That is, simply give your full attention to what you are doing at that given moment. The benefits you will gain by doing this include, you will notice that your time is a lot more meaningful and productive, you will sleep better at night and accomplish more at work, your conversations will be more meaningful to both yourself and whomever you are talking to, and you will be able to notice a lot more opportunities that arise because you are tuned in to the present moment. So the next time you engage in conversation with someone, be sure to give them your undivided attention by controlling your thoughts and FOCUSING in on listening and remember to be here now in the present moment and they will be sure to show you the same respect in return and share more opportunities with you.

This especially applies to dating. Your date will feel more appreciated because of your ability to completely focus in on them each moment you are with them and in return will respect you more as a result. Not to mention, they will be a lot more interested in you as a result of being in control of your thoughts and learning how to "be here now in the present moment". Even if an extremely beautiful person walks by or tries to flirt with you, continue to "be here now in the present moment" and give your undivided attention to the person you are with while engaged in a conversation or activity. The rewards will be well worth your effort. Remember, the past is history, the present is a gift, and the future has not happened yet.

When we stop to carefully think about this concept of being here now in the present moment, we realize that the present is really all we have any control over. Once you realize and accept this fact, you will be capable of accomplishing some pretty amazing things. For example, you know from previous chapters that "small commitments lead to larger commitments", right? Well knowing this, you can apply the "be here now in the present moment" concept to give a potential date you complete undivided attention to gradually move to the next level and/or step of actually dating that person. Perhaps you have only gotten as far as engaging in conversation with someone you would like to start dating.

Knowing that small commitments lead to larger commitments, you must realize that you have taken the first big step towards reaching your goal of dating this person. The fact that the person has even acknowledged you and has agreed to engage in conversation with you lets you know that you have opened the door to slowly proceed to the next step. However long this process takes will depend on the individuals and circumstances involved. The fact is however, by being here now in the present moment while engaged in conversation with your potential date, you want to convey to them through body language, facial expressions, eye contact, and language that you are interested in them. From this point you want to move very slowly to the next step and accomplish the goal of asking them out.

The best time and way to accomplish this is after you are certain your potential date feels comfortable being engaged in a conversation with you. Once this is certain, you want to proceed slowly by asking them in a very subtle way using something similar to one of the following questions. "Would you mind if we get together tomorrow morning / afternoon / evening for about 30 minutes to enjoy a cup of coffee or tea and spend some time to get to know each other a little better?", or "Would you mind if we get together tomorrow morning / afternoon / evening for about 30 minutes to get some desert and coffee or tea and spend some time to get to know each other a little better?". You could ask about dinner if you feel comfortable but remember that may seem a little too presumptive to some people.

By asking them to meet with you over a cup of coffee or tea for about 30 minutes and spending some time to get to know each other a little better, accomplishes the following:

1. It allows you to transition over from just being involved in conversation to spending more time together.

2. It tests the waters to see if the other person is interested in pursuing the next step with you.

3. It lets the other person feel comfortable that you are only meeting for coffee or tea, no strings attached.

4. It establishes how long you plan on spending time together.

5. It establishes the main FOCUS of why you want to spend time together.

They will either say "yes" or "no". If they say something like "I will try to meet you tomorrow...", (immediately remember from the previous chapter, Try Implies Failure!), then say to them, "you know it sounds like you may be busy tomorrow. Rather than trying to meet me for coffee or tea tomorrow, can you be certain to meet me on Thursday?" At this point they have to level with you and let you know that "yes, Thursday is a good day to meet up with you" or they will have to be honest and let you know that they do not feel like it would be a good idea for both of you to pursue getting to know each other better.

Either way, you are not left hanging or wondering what is going on!? You know where you stand with this person at that moment. Above all, proceed very slowly. People get intimidated or clam up if you attempt to move too quickly. Take your time, get to know the person as much as you can and then decide if you want to pursue it further. If so, think about how you are going to make them feel good about meeting up with you? In other words, what would compel them to want to meet up with you? Are you very attractive, very nice, very polite, very smart, common interests, love art, love museums, rich? You get the picture, now give them a compelling reason to want to meet up with you and proceed very slowly and remember, "be here now in the present moment".

If it works out GREAT! If not, don't give up, be persistent! Either take a step back and re-strategize another game plan or move on with your life to finding somebody else that matches your criteria. The key here is to remain friendly, courteous, and professional no matter how things end up. You never know who they know.

Chapter 32

"With Every Loss There Is A Gain"

With Every Loss There Is A Gain - It may be difficult to recognize while you are still emotionally attached to the loss you have experienced. As time passes by, you will slowly begin to understand the reason or purpose for your loss and as you begin to understand the reason, you will begin to realize that while you may have lost something, you really have gained something in place of that loss. Maybe you have lost a loved one due to death in your family, a spouse due to divorce, a dating partner to someone else, a secure job or maybe you have lost a limb in a car accident. Whatever your loss is, take time to grieve and remember that there was a purpose or reason for your loss.

After you have accepted your loss and realize that there was a purpose or reason fro your loss and pulled yourself back together, you will slowly begin to notice the gain that came about as a result of your loss. Perhaps it is in the form of strength, or courage, or confidence, or an acceptance, or an understanding, or a new beginning, maybe it is a better opportunity, a lesson learned, or an opportunity to start fresh all over again. Whatever your gain is, it was meant specifically just for you and only you will come to learn what that gain is through the passage of time. Remember, whatever does not kill us only makes us stronger! Take your new found strength and do something positive and productive with it for yourself and for everyone else around you.

So the next time that you meet someone or go out on a date and things do not work out for you, just remember that with every loss there is a gain. Take the time you need to recover and accept your loss, realize that there was a reason or purpose for your loss, and begin to find your new found strength. Once you have your new found strength, keep your eyes open and your mind alert because your gain is waiting for you directly ahead. All you need to do is show up and embrace it. Chances are, you will be much more prepared and ready this time.

Chapter 33:

"Underlying Reasons"

Underlying Reasons – One of the biggest misconceptions that I have found in relationships is that for the most part, people involved in a new relationship really do not know and understand each other that well. To complicate this situation, the two people begin to form habits and patterns for one reason or another as the relationship progresses. In the early stages of the relationship, things aren't too bad and the couple is very forgiving towards each other. As the relationship progresses and the couple becomes more relaxed and comfortable being in front of each other, they begin to settle into their old and habitual ways whether good or bad. As more and more time passes, if the couple learns to openly and honestly communicate effectively with each other from the very beginning of their relationship, they should be able to enjoy a long and prosperous relationship for the most part with an occasional argument here and there.

However, if the couple fails to learn to openly and honestly communicate effectively with each other starting in the very beginning of their relationship, their relationship will either be short lived for a number of different reasons or full of arguments, frustration, and challenges until the couple both agree to either seek counseling and learn to unconditionally accept the other for who they are and forgive each other for not being completely honest and admit to their contribution of problems up to that point in their relationship. Some of the underlying reasons that couples may fail to openly and honestly communicate with each other include fear of rejection, fear of loss, and fear of failure, fear of being misunderstood, fear of past problems or mistakes, or fear of current situations.

However, the real problem begins after the couple has been together for awhile and decided to stick together and work things out and have not yet made a conscious decision to seek counseling to uncover their underlying problems. The reason that this time of their relationship can be such a problem is because one or both people may begin to experience feelings of being misunderstood by the other or may feel a lack of adequate understanding by the other. When this occurs, one or both people in this relationship will begin acting or behaving certain ways that seem to be triggered by certain experiences in their relationship. For example, one person may decide that they are so frustrated in the relationship that they do not want to communicate with the other; meanwhile, the other person may decide to begin drinking alcohol or taking drugs because in their mind they feel misunderstood about why the other person will not communicate with them. This is kind of their self-justification acting out.

Meanwhile, the person that does not want to communicate is convinced that their partner has a drinking problem not realizing that one of the main underlying reasons for their drinking problem is because they decided not to communicate with the drinking partner. I used drinking in this particular example because I personally experienced this same exact problem with my current wife. She did not want to communicate with me because of how we started off our relationship with a lack of open and honest communication and I decided to begin drinking more often because I felt misunderstood and that she did not want to communicate with me. In place of drinking, some people resort to sex, drugs, you name it. Fortunately, we decided we loved each other too much and wanted to save and improve our marriage relationship and sought marriage counseling as a result.

So please remember, when you first start off in a relationship, take some time to explain to your partner the importance of open and honest communication and how it can help your relationship blossom and turn into something beautiful. Remember also that there are underlying reasons why people act certain ways or do certain things. Instead of immediately dismissing someone as having a mental problem or looking down on them as an alcoholic, take a step back and ask yourself what could be the underlying reason for someone acting this way or doing such an odd thing? Chances are with a little bit of digging and a few sincere questions; you will allow this person to open up and uncover the real reason that is causing them to act in such a way. Life works in very funny and mysterious ways, so by taking the time to learn, understand, and help someone out by uncovering and bringing to the surface their underlying reasons, you will be doing this person huge favor because it allows them a pathway to get themselves back on track. Besides, who knows, the next time around, that person that needs help could be you!

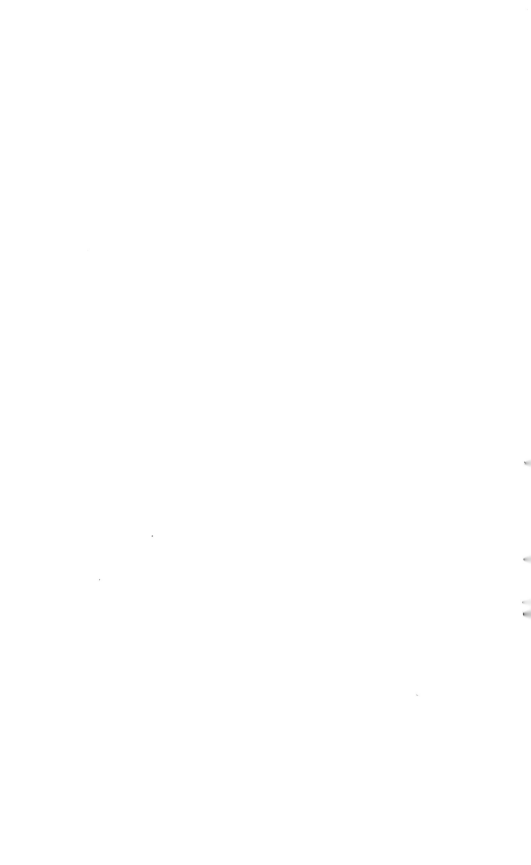

Chapter 34:

"Responsibility"

Responsibility – I know this may seem obvious to most people so please continue reading this chapter and hopefully you will learn something new here. Most people relate responsibility to paying their bills, performing well at their job, doing their chores, and pulling their own weight. While these are certainly some of the requirements of responsibility and being a responsible person, there is a lot more to it than just that, especially when it comes to relationships. In a relationship, being responsible also means accepting blame for something that went wrong, not pointing fingers at someone else, accepting the consequences of your actions, making sure that you understand what is being said by someone else, and making sure that everyone else understands what you are saying and accepting the consequences if not.

The immediate benefits that you will gain out of being more responsible, include:

1. Having a much better understanding of what people say and mean.
2. Likewise, other people will better understand what you are saying and what you mean.
3. People will respect you more because you are not quick to point fingers and try to blame someone else rather you are a person that accepts full responsibility.
4. The opposite sex will really take notice and like you a lot better for this one reason alone.

5. You will notice that you have fewer mistakes because you are more careful with your decisions and actions by realizing that there are now consequences to all of your actions.

6. People will become more attracted to you and you will gain a better reputation for being someone who accepts responsibility.

Being from Singapore, my wife for example sometimes has a little bit of difficulty explaining herself to someone else or understanding the meaning that someone else is presenting to her. Often times when I notice this I will step in and interpret either what she is attempting to convey to someone or explain the meaning of what someone else is attempting to convey to her. I do this for good reason; I have a vested interest in my wife's health and livelihood. I feel that if I can help her explain or understand something more accurately the way that it was intended, it will help save her time and frustration. Though she may not agree at that moment that I am helping her, she soon realizes that my efforts of helping to clarify things for her own understanding and helping to explain her point of view to others helps to make her life better and safer and helps her to better understand the world around her.

This is not to say that my wife is not intelligent nor capable of understanding or explaining herself, far from the truth, she is actually very intelligent. I just happen to be very good at understanding what other people are saying and what they really mean by what they are saying. I'm also very good at being able to understand and explain her meaning to them. This is another example of being responsible by helping out to make sure that my wife is protected by making sure there is no misunderstanding in what she is saying as well as what is being said to her. You can accomplish this yourself simply by taking what is being said and rephrasing it in the form of a question with the meaning that you perceived to be true. If your translation is not accurate, they will tell you what they really meant.

For example: While at a business networking function, my wife was approached by a business owner wanting information about her company. Her understanding of what was being said is that the business owner wanted to use her services for hiring new people. Naturally, she was excited at the fact that someone was asking about her business and the services she offers. As I listened in, I understood the business owner to be asking for information on what she charges for her recruiting services because he has several new employees to hire and wanted to get some perspective on what it would cost him to go through a recruiting firm.

Granted, he might be interested in using her services after he feels comfortable with the fee she charges however at this point in the conversation all he wanted was some pricing and information. She had interpreted it to mean that the business owner wanted to use her company for placing these new candidates. After explaining to her what he really said and meant, she then proceeded to explain to him how her fee schedule works. Needless to say, he could not afford to pay for her employment recruiting services after understanding her fee schedule. After going through that experience, you can only imagine that from now on, she makes sure that she understands exactly what a business owner is asking for as well as how much they can afford and is now more responsible in making sure she fully understands both sides of the conversation.

So the next time you are out on a date or meet someone new for the very first time, decide to take the responsibility to make sure that you fully understand both the words and meaning of what the other person is really saying to you as well as take responsibility to make sure they understand what you are saying to them. That way, there is very little room for margin of error and at the end of the night, you and your date will feel like they are with someone that really and truly understands the responsibility of properly communicating with other people and each other. Remember, it is ultimately up to you to CHOOSE to make sure that everyone you speak to completely understands what you are saying and what you mean by what you are saying.

Chapter 35:

"Diversions"

Diversions – Look out for diversions because they are used to mislead you and throw you off track! They come from out of nowhere and are used to completely change the topic or subject of discussion. Most people use them to escape from a particular conversation or question that they feel uncomfortable about. What makes diversions really tricky is that the person using the diversion will start off by answering your question and then completely switch to another topic in mid-conversation that has absolutely no relevance to the information you were concerned with or questioning them about. Diversions are designed take your mind off of the information you were after and focuses your attention and/or concern over to a completely different topic and is usually done without you even realizing it just happened. People will also use diversions to transition from one topic to another.

The main reasons that most people use diversions are because either they feel uncomfortable about the conversation they are involved in, they are trying to hide something from you, they figure that by creating a diversion they can temporarily escape telling you the truth, they feel that they are protecting you from exposure to certain information, or they want to escape from the feeling of being put in the spotlight. Whatever the reason is that people choose to create diversions, you need to be able to identify that a diversion was just created and whether or not the information that you are after is important enough to bring their attention back to your question or topic of discussion. You need to also realize that if enough time goes by after the diversion was created; chances are very strong that you will not have the opportunity to bring their attention back to the topic of discussion or question at hand.

The reality is that we have all fallen victim to diversions in one form or another and probably encounter at least one diversion if not more every single day. Although diversions can have both a positive and negative impact on us, most of the time, people will use diversions for their own self benefit. What this means is that the diversion they used was probably used use to have a negative impact on us rather than on them. Some good examples of this include using diversions to delay paying back money you owe, returning something you borrowed, honoring your commitment to someone, being on time, accepting responsibility, and the list goes on and on.

So the next time you ask someone a specific question or are looking for a specific answer, make sure you do not fall victim to someone else's diversion tactics. If you notice that they were able to create a diversion and change the topic of discussion, quickly bring the conversation back to the topic that you were concerned with before the diversion was created. For example let us say that John owes you money that you loaned him over a month ago. You finally manage to catch up with John at the shopping mall and ask John if he has the money you loaned him last month. John immediately begins telling you all about the problems he is having financially and that he just started a new job with all kinds of nice benefits and vacation time and then quickly asks you, by the way, how are your parents are doing? Immediately realize that John just attempted to create a diversion from the money he owes you by asking you about your parents.

You could reply back to John and say. John, my parents are doing wonderful and I'm really happy to hear that your new job is going so well, so please tell me again when I'm supposed to be repaid the money that you owe me? Another example would be if you wanted to go out on a date with someone new you just met. You start up a conversation and begin getting to know this person that you just met. Suddenly, you pop the question by asking if they would like to go out for dinner tomorrow night. They start off by saying that their parents just got in to town and that they haven't seen them for 5 years and that there is so much to catch up on and bla, bla, bla. You could reply by saying…"that is so wonderful, I am so happy for you, so does this mean that we are going out for dinner tomorrow night with or without your parents?" This way you can thank them and show them respect for the other information that they diverted you over to, and at the same time politely bring the conversation back in to focus.

As you can see, it is very easy for someone to throw you off track or suddenly change topics in just a split second. If you are none the wiser, then you will fall victim every time it happens. At some point there comes a time when monetary value involved. If you are alert enough to catch the diversions when they happen, not only will you come out ahead, you will also keep your loss of time and money to a minimum. So remember, keep FOCUSED on the end result and listen out carefully for diversions and bring the conversation back in to focus if things get off track.

Chapter 36:

"Count To 10"

Count To 10 – Even better, count 24 to 48 hours. That is 24 to 48 hours before you reply or respond back to someone who has delivered you an insult or some devastating news. The purpose for this is that my experience has led me to understand that by taking at least this much time to reply or respond back to someone about such news, empowers you with all the right and possible answers that otherwise would come across as an answer from someone who was immature or irresponsible. Think about it! How many times have you been in a situation whereby someone has said something to you that either offended you or caught you off guard and in retaliation you immediately fired off a response that you later regretted?

I know this too well from personal experience in dealing with my current wife who had a habit of throwing up diversions and trying to capitalize on the heat of the moment to prove how wrong I am about a certain topic or subject. What I have learned is that if I take between 24 to 48 hours to give my reply or response, not only have I had enough time to completely think things through, more importantly, I have allowed myself enough time to craft the right and most justified answer to her accusation which in turn enables her to realize that I am really a good person with good intentions looking out for her best interest and that she totally misunderstood me as both a person and a spouse in the heat of the moment.

Since learning and implementing this important rule of "Counting to 10", we now both have the utmost respect for each other and know our limits and boundaries and since we both ultimately just want to be in love with each other, we both do our very best and usually CHOOSE to "Count to 10" to let things cool down before replying to each other. This allows the situation to cool down and allows us to amicably move past the situation and resume loving and caring for each other.

So the next time you find yourself caught up in the heat of the moment, remember to "Count to 10" and in the process think of how you would like to see situation get resolved and how the outcome is ultimately going to affect your relationship. Some people just want to argue while most want to quickly move past the arguments and resume loving each other.

Chapter 37:

"Whatever Does Not Kill You"

Whatever Does Not Kill You – You know the old saying…"whatever does not kill you will only make you stronger", right? Well I know for a fact that I have become a much stronger person, and so can you. With each day that passes we experience situations that really put us to the test and when we look back, we see how much we have learned, how far we have come, and how strong we have become in the process. Can you remember a point in your life when you were first confronted with a situation that seemed almost impossible? Chances are, you were either thinking to yourself, I am not strong enough to do this or I do not know how I am ever going to get through this, right? Well look how far you have come! Now when confronted with that same task, chances are, you do not even stop to think about it, you just simply do it with ease.

The same is true for everyone else and with every new situation you will ever encounter. You either already know how to handle the situation because you have experienced it before or it seems totally foreign to you because you have never experienced it before. Either way, you have a task in front of you that has to be dealt with. So knowing that "whatever does not kill you only makes you stronger", learn to accept and embrace new situations that you are confronted with from now on. By doing this and realizing that you only become stronger as a result, makes you a much better prepared person for any unexpected situation or opportunity that arises.

So remember that the next time you are confronted with being rejected for a date, or turned down for an offer to get to know someone better, or make an attempt to advance your relationship to the next stage, remember that "whatever does not kill you" will only make you stronger. Learn from these experiences and carry those lessons forward to your next relationship attempt and continue bringing those lessons forward in your attempt to have the ideal relationship and continue being persistent and determined to find that special relationship. It is definitely out there, it is just difficult to find sometimes. This leads us into our next successful psychological principle.

Chapter 38:

"Fail Forward Fast"

Fail Forward Fast – Almost everyone you talk to will equate doing something wrong or performing a certain task incorrectly with being a failure. I completely disagree! I feel that you are only a failure if you quit after doing something wrong. A true winner will go back again and again and again until they learn to perform their task successfully. That is the definition of a true winner.

You now know that "whatever does not kill you will only make you stronger", right? Well then why not step out of your comfort zone and take a few chances doing something new and different? After all, doesn't your life get boring from doing the same things over and over again? There is certainly no evolution in that. Try the following exercise for a change. Purposely choose to put yourself in a new or different situation or environment than what you are now used to being in and remain completely open-minded. Do this with the understanding that you are going to attempt something new and are going to learn to "Fail Forward Fast".

This means that whatever new task you have decided to embark on, whatever it is, realize and accept that you may feel uncomfortable at first doing it, everyone does. Also have the open-mindedness and understanding that most likely you are going to make mistakes and in the process are going to learn to "Fail Forward Fast". This is the moment you want to learn to accept and embrace your newfound sense of excitement and nervousness. Since you may not know exactly what you are doing, realize that there can only be two possibilities. Either you performed your new task the right way or the wrong way. Either way you win because you took a new step forward.

Failing forward fast means deciding that you are going to accomplish something new and charging forward to do it regardless of whether you know how to do it or not. The benefit comes from your realization that even if you do not know exactly what you are doing, and end up doing the wrong thing, you will quickly learn from your mistakes, the right way of performing your new task. Since you know that the chances are great that you are going to make a mistake and have accepted this already in advance, let nothing hold you back or get in your way from going thru with your new task to completion whatever the outcome may be.

Once you have finished your new task to the best of your ability, quickly analyze whether you performed your new task the right way or decide if you made some mistakes and performed your new task the wrong way? If you performed your new task correctly the first time, then you deserve a Congratulations! If you performed your new task incorrectly, or made some mistakes, then realize that you are now one step closer to understanding how to perform your new task correctly the next time. Continue this process of "failing forward fast" until you perform your new task correctly.

This sense of knowledge and understanding about "Failing Forward Fast" can be applied in almost every area of your life. Think of some new ways you can now begin using this knowledge and understanding at your job, with your family, in your relationships, it is endless. I recently used this concept while attempting to cook for my wife. She was amazed that I even made the attempt. Of course she was very understanding of the fact that my cooking did not taste as good as her cooking. Nonetheless, she still thanked me for trying and made some very good suggestions on what I could do next time to make it taste even better.

Now that you understand the basic concept, let me share a great example of how you can use this concept to meet other people. I used this new concept to try out a new pick up line that actually worked the first time I used it. I was at a local bar going towards the men's bathroom and saw this very beautiful lady coming out of the women's bathroom towards me. The instant I saw her, I felt like

I had been hit in the chest and knocked back about ten feet from her beauty! She was absolutely stunning! Her presence had such an impact on me, I actually had trouble breathing for a few minutes. I made my way to the bathroom and quickly went back out to my seat. I saw her standing in the middle of the floor with three other guys swarming around her like bees talking to her.

I instantly thought to myself, "I don't even stand a chance". Then my friend noticed me looking at her and sulking and said to me "go over and talk to her". I was nervous and frozen. I could not even stand up because my legs were so shaky. Finally, without warning, my friend pushed me over towards her. He pushed me so hard, that I bumped into her and the three other guys. She quickly turned around and looked at me with concern, and I had to apologize for bumping into her. She quickly accepted my apology and without hesitation I decided this is my moment to "Fail Forward Fast"! She was either going to say "yes" or "no".

While I had her attention, I immediately said to her..."I cannot help but notice how beautiful you look today...I do not have some fancy line to tell you like...I want to show you the stars or anything like that, however I would like to ask if you would be interested in going out for some coffee or tea sometime and getting to know each other a little better where it is not so crowded and noisy?" Amazingly, she said "sure, that would be just fine". You can only imagine how excited I was for the next twenty-four hours straight! I could not get her out of my mind! I immediately thought to myself, I succeeded in "Failing Forward Fast" by using a pick up line that I had never used before simply by CHOOSING to make the effort!

I have also had the opposite experience happen to me before and had to go back and refine what I was saying and how I was saying it, to make it sound more genuine and convincing. The fact is simple, if you do not CHOOSE to make the attempt you will never know what the outcome could have been. Instead of worrying about getting all of the details just right and perfect and procrastinating, leap forward with an open mind and embrace the fact that you are going to "Fail Forward Fast" and learn the right way of performing the new task at hand through the process of doing it wrong. Above all else, remember that you are only a failure if you give up after not succeeding. As long as you continue making the attempt to do things better the next time by learning from your mistakes, then you are by all definitions considered at success.

So the next time you are faced with a new or unique situation that involves stepping out of your comfort zone, gather your courage and remember to "fail forward fast" and learn from your mistakes quickly and keep carrying those experiences forward to your next attempt and so on until you have finally discovered your ideal relationship.

Chapter 39:

"90% Of The Time"

90% Of The Time – 90% of the time you can accomplish at least two things at once simply by taking an extra moment or two and asking yourself and thinking about what else needs to be done or taken care of before you set out to accomplish your first task? For example, since you are already going into the freezer to get some ice for your water, you could also take out the chicken from the freezer that needs to be defrosted for dinner. I have learned over the years that by taking a few extra seconds to simply think through what I am about to do, I can almost always think of something else that I can accomplish at the same time or within the same trip which ultimately allows me to get more things done in less time.

This can work especially well for enhancing your relationships. For example, if you are already going to the store to get groceries, pick up a nice greeting card while you are there, or a bottle of wine, or a small bouquet of flowers, or even a plant. Think about the little things. You will be surprised at how much of an impact these little things have on improving the quality of your relationships. When you really stop and think about it, isn't it the small things in life that other people do for us that we remember the most? Then certainly it is all of the small things that you do for someone else that will help keep that person attracted to you. So the next time you have to go somewhere or do something, take a few extra seconds to remember about "90% Of The Time", and ask yourself..."what else can I accomplish or take care of at the same time that will help enhance my life and my relationships?"

This principle also applies to your personal self by being able to get more things accomplished for yourself in less time, hassle, and expense. It also applies to your job functions. What better way for you to make yourself more productive and valuable in your boss's eyes than by being able to get more accomplished in the same or less amount of time? Just by simply taking a few extra seconds to think through what else needs to be done or accomplished in the direction you are setting out in? You will be absolutely amazed after a while at how much more you cam get accomplished and how much more enhanced your relationships become as a result.

So the next time you are involved in discovering a new relationship or going out on a date with your existing relationship, remember that "90% of the time" you can do something additional or extra to help improve and strengthen your relationship, and most of the time it can be something small or inexpensive that can make all the difference. Just CHOOSE to put your mind to it.

Chapter 40

"Gut Feelings"

Gut Feelings – This is one lesson I had to learn the hard way. I find it amazing how when we as humans discover something new that works in our lives, we develop habits of not continuing with our newly found discovery and soon we are back on our old paths again wondering why we are not making progress. I learned a long time ago from my father to always trust your gut feelings or gut instincts as some people call it. For me this principle worked fine while I was still living at home, but as soon as moved out, it seemed this principle no longer applied to me. So I thought. I soon realized that I was making a lot of decisions and taking actions against my gut feelings.

Several years later I realized that this was one of my biggest mistakes. Have you ever been in a situation whereby you were about to make a purchase and a voice inside of you keeps saying do not purchase it and you start have twisted knot feeling in your stomach? Well, that is your gut feelings or gut instincts talking to you. I found myself losing lots of money, being taken advantage of, and not enjoying the types of relationships that I wanted.

Believe it or not, those gut feelings are warnings that are designed to protect you. The weird part that I later discovered about these gut feelings is that most of the time, our gut feelings protect us from things that we do not yet know about. I'll repeat this one more time. "Most of the time, our gut feelings protect us from things that we do not yet know about." Sound kind of spooky? The fact is, our brain thinks in logic and our heart senses in feelings. Combine those two with who you really are, your spirit, and suddenly you have the uncanny ability to emit certain feelings designed to protect yourself from things that are about to happen or have not yet happened.

Either way, learn to tune in to these feelings because they can ultimately end up saving your life. I know this for a fact because my gut feelings have helped save my life on at least three different occasions. This especially applies to relationships with other people and most definitely people that you do not know quite well enough yet to let your guard down. Whatever the situation might be, never feel embarrassed about backing away from someone or something that is about to happen especially if your gut feeling is telling you that something does not seem right. Better stated, never go against your gut feelings. If you do go against your gut feelings, 99.9% of the time, you will end up wishing that you had not.

So the next time you find yourself in a situation whereby your gut feelings are speaking to you, listen to them! It could be the one time that ends up saving your life.

Chapter: 41

"First Impressions"

First Impressions – First impressions have a lasting affect and can sometimes last a lifetime. This truth applies to all areas of your life and especially with your job, your social life AND your dating life. You have heard of the old cliché'..."you only get one chance to make a good first impression", right? Because your future relationships are at stake here, we want to take it a step further. Instead of making a good first impression, why not make a great first impression? After all, my experience has proven to me time and again that it is the small little details that most of us overlook that help persuade or entice someone else's decision.

Think about this very carefully for a moment especially if you are going after a certain individual and there is competition involved. Sometimes it is very difficult for the individual you are going after to make a decision about whom they would rather be with. So by making a conscientious effort to make great first impression, could prove to be the deciding factor for the individual you are going after. It may sound petty, but believe me I have been in this situation before and have both won and lost the person I was going after when competition was involved. When I reflect back over the wins and losses, almost every time I can think of, the final decision ended up being the result of the first impression.

If you are sincerely interested in dating a person you know or have recently met and have not formally introduced yourself yet. Bare in mind that your initial introduction, actions, words, and body language will ultimately be the deciding factor as to whether the other person will like you or not. In fact studies show that you have less than 30 seconds to prove yourself before the other person forms an initial opinion about you. That does not give you a lot of time so you better practice in front of a mirror before making the attempt.

Make sure you know exactly what you want to say, how you want to convey your introduction, what you want your body language to look like, what you want your facial expressions to look like, and a clear mental picture of what you want the end result to look like. For example, when I would make an initial introduction, I wanted to say something very positive and uplifting while not sounding too saucy. At the same time, I wanted to present myself in a confident manner with good posture and yet not too close as to invade the other persons space or aura. I especially wanted to be smiling and appear genuine and the mental picture in my mind was one of me and the other person already being out on a nice romantic date with both of us extremely happy.

As I said earlier, sometimes it works out that way and sometimes it does not. If for some reason you blow your first impression and things do not work out the way you want them to, do not throw in the towel just yet. However, you need to make a long and serious decision about whether you are willing to do whatever it takes to win this person over. You obviously need to be intent on staying with this person for a long time to make the next attempt worth your time and effort. If after a long debate with yourself you finally decide that you want to be with this person for the rest of your life and there is no doubt that this is the right person for you, then prepare to pay very close attention on how to win this person over.

The very first thing you have to do is except the fact that you may never end up being with this person. The next thing you need to do is determine what price you are willing to pay and how much are you willing to sacrifice to win this person over? The very next thing you need to do is determine what is your plan of action going to be to keep this person in love with you once you win them over? Keep in mind, almost everybody can put on a great first or second impression, but what you do AFTER THAT determines who you really are. Are you a fun, loving, outgoing, adventurous type of person, or are you a quiet, reclusive, shy type of person? This is why it is vitally important to the success of your continued relationship and happiness that you have a plan of action to keep the relationship alive and vibrant!

If you are prepared for all of this and want a second chance at making a great first impression, then here is what you need to know and how you need to proceed. First, get up enough nerve to go back and meet with the other person and sincerely explain to them that when you first introduced yourself or attempted to convey your feelings, you were so impressed with their beauty, charisma, smile, etc. (whatever it was that impressed you) and that it made you completely nervous and unable to function in front of them. You do this for three very good reasons. One, it gives you the opportunity to pay the other person a sincere compliment. Two, it shows the other person your human side and makes them feel impressed that you felt nervous in their presence. Three, it humbles you in their presence so they can see who you really are and what you are really made of. This is the real person they want to meet and know and be with.

This is where the relationship starts. All you can really ask for is the opportunity for the other person to allow you to express your feelings towards them. From there it is up to the other person to respond in a way that they feel is appropriate for them. If after being successful in your second attempt to make a great impression, and the other person agrees to date you, and you go out to dinner or you go out for a cup of coffee, etc.. Then NOW is when you really have your work cut out for yourself. Because from that moment on, you NOW have to keep selling yourself to the other person every single day that you are the right person for them based on their expectations. They may not tell you this directly verbatim, but trust me an evaluation is constantly being made every day to determine or reinforce whether or not you are the right person or not. So stay on top of your game and do the very best you can to make it a fun and loving relationship. Most likely you are doing or thinking the same exact thing about the other person every day..."is this the right person for me?"

The only saving grace that you may have going for yourself is that since you are already involved in the relationship, the other person will hopefully feel some sense of loyalty and be willing to forgive and forget a number of your mistakes provided that you have not caused any direct harm that cannot be overcome. The important lesson here is, never allow yourself to become complacent in your relationship. Always think about and look for ways to keep your relationship evolving, exciting, and fun. Since you cannot force someone to want to stay with you, figure out how you can make them want to be with you on their own free will.

So the next time you are faced with the opportunity of making a first impression, take your opportunity seriously and make the most of it. Even if things do not work out for the best, you will be remembered as someone that always puts their best foot forward.

Chapter 42:

"Voice Inflections"

Voice Inflections – Voice inflections play a very important part in the realm of the subconscious as well as the conscious and in understanding body language.

The subconscious is affected by voice inflections in that as you are speaking, the tone, pace, and pitch of your voice is constantly sending data to the subconscious mind of the listener. This data is translated into feelings based on past experiences, and first impressions and is brought to the conscious mind in the form of a perception. This happens so quickly that you do not realize that this process just happened. Therefore it is very important to constantly monitor how your voice is being perceived when you speak. The good news is that we have the ability to make adjustments on how our voice sounds, and is perceived by changing our voice inflections. This may sound a little far fetched, but believe you me, everything you do and say; and how you do it and how you say it, is creating an impression on the people that are listening to you. The fact is, is that these impressions are being processed and happening so fast, that you do not realize it is happening.

Body language is affected by voice inflections in that as you are speaking to someone, they are constantly monitoring your body language to ensure that they completely understand exactly what you are saying. If your voice inflections do not match your body language then you may be sending mixed signals and possibly confusing your listeners. For example, if your voice inflection is of a soft, gentle speaker and your body language is showing crossed arms, while your posture is standing rigidly straight, you would confuse your listeners into thinking more about how you are actually feeling rather than listening to what you saying. Therefore, your voice inflections and body language must be in sync with each other in order for your listeners to completely understand your body language and listen to what you are saying. The best way to keep this in check is to consciously think about your voice inflections matching up along with your body language.

Above all, remember that your voice inflections, body language, words, actions, facial expressions, and attitudes are all being assessed faster than you realize and that the ongoing data is being compiled and stored in the subconscious mind which is why the perception of the relationship is constantly changing and evolving. As a result, you must be conscious of all these at all times while you are communicating.

Chapter 43:

"Do It Now"

Do It Now – This is probably one of the most important lessons I have ever learned. That is to "do it now". Do what now, you ask? Whatever it is that needs to be done. "Do it NOW or it won't get done!" Seize the opportunity!

Before I learned about this important lesson, I would always say..."I will take care of this problem tomorrow instead of doing it now". What I discovered was that tomorrow came and I kept putting off handling the problem until it got so bad that I was forced to deal with it. The reality is that everyone puts off doing things they know they need to do. Very few people actually make the effort to "do it now" and get it over and done with. What I learned from taking the initiative to "do it now" is that the things I needed to accomplish were getting done a lot quicker. Additionally, I felt better about myself for doing it, and I began to get recognized by others as someone who can get the job done.

So if you find yourself in a situation whereby you are attracted to someone that is available, do not put it off until tomorrow or the next time, "DO IT NOW", go up to them and let them know that you find them very attractive and would like to invite them out to either dinner, or coffee, or tea, the park, wherever, just "do it now" and remember to make a great first impression. Only one of two things can happen. Either they say sure I will go out with you, or they say no. If they say "no", refer back to what you learned in the lesson "Obviously You Have A Reason" because you at least want to make the attempt to find out what their reason is for saying "no". Either way, learn to "do it now" and have no regrets about something you wish you had of done. Besides, life is too short to be procrastinating and putting things off.

Chapter 44:

"A Numbers Game"

A Numbers Game – You have heard of the old cliché, "it is a numbers game", right? Well guess what? It is true! Everything from sales, to sports, to dating is a numbers game. Ask enough people out and someone is going to say "yes". They may not be the ideal person you have been dreaming of, but if you ask enough people out, someone is going to say "yes". Learn the important lessons taught in this book and your standards of whom you ask out will increase as a result. That is because you will have a much better understanding at how to go about finding the right type of person and you will know how to make yourself more attractive to that person. Most importantly, you will learn how to keep yourself attractive to that special person.

Towards the beginning of this book I explained that before you set your heart on dating and meeting people through the Internet, the Grocery Store, the Mall etc., I feel it is extremely important that you first learn some psychology and some very important life lessons about dating and human beings that you can begin applying and using from this moment forward in all of your relationships. This includes your family, co-workers, existing friends, new friends, lovers...everybody.

The reason I suggest this is because it is easy to teach someone how to be more attractive to others. However, teaching someone about the underlying psychology that is inevitably involved in every relationship is not so easy. Therefore, you should have a very strong understanding about the human psychology as it relates to relationships, which I have summarized in this book, before setting out to get involved in a serious relationship and / or marriage. Trust me, you will be very grateful that you took the time to read, understand, learn and do your due diligence. After all, you want to make certain that you have the very best shot at impressing that special someone when you finally find them, right?

So now that you have taken time to read, learn, and understand the psychology of human beings as it relates to relationships, learned how to put your best foot forward, how to better identify problems in the relationship, how to better present yourself and communicate more effectively, you should be about ready to start playing the numbers game. I am going to share with you how I personally went about finding my wife playing the numbers game. Before I do, please allow me to set the stage for what prompted me to make this decision at this moment in my life.

On July 15, 2000, I took a very attractive young lady out to dinner with some of my very close friends that I have known for almost 20 years. While at dinner, I had the unfortunate experience of learning that my date loves to run her mouth and dominate every conversation she gets involved in. After about 30 minutes, I noticed some of my friends glancing over at me and rolling their eyes. I knew at this point that they too were being completely annoyed by my date. The straw that broke the camels back was when my date said something inappropriate about me that she later clarified with me after we left the restaurant.

While driving back to my house, she kept talking, and talking, and talking. Finally, I asked her to please just sit there and be silent for five minutes. After about 30 seconds passed, she began talking again. At this moment, I had made up my mind that I did not want to see her anymore. When I pulled into my driveway, I asked her to please just go home and let her know that I did not want to date her anymore. Full of anger about how she presented herself and acted in front of my closest friends, I decided right then and there that I was going to follow my passion no matter what. That is to find a beautiful Asian woman that could cook good, looked good, had a great attitude, and was in involved in Information Technology sales.

Honestly, at this point I did not care what part of the world she lived in because I was determined to meet her. So I immediately logged on to the Internet and began browsing for Asian females that fit into my specifications and no limitations on the Country. Amazingly, I retrieved 53 online profiles around the world, most of them living somewhere in Asia, that met my criteria. After reading through each one, I narrowed the list down to 25. Out of the 25, one in particular really caught my attention. In fact I actually felt as if she jumped out of the monitor towards me the second I saw her picture online. Not allowing myself to be distracted and not getting my hopes up too much, I sent the following email to all 25 of them.

"Hi, I saw your personal profile online and could not help but notice how attractive you are. I am a single white male living in the U.S. and looking for a serious relationship that will eventually lead to marriage. It is your beauty that caught my eye, but it is your heart that will keep me. If you are searching for someone that is serious, please reply back and allow us to get to know each other a little better. Sincerely, Robert Davenport"

All total, I received 15 different replies from the 25 I sent out. However, within 30 minutes of sending out my email, I received the first reply who happened to be the person that I felt jump out of the monitor towards me. I was shocked and nervous and scared all at once. I knew this was my opportunity to finally meet the girl of my dreams. She replied back asking me to chat with her on AOL Instant Messenger. After 15 minutes of chatting, she asked if I would mind if she called me. Of course I did not mind...except for the fact that I was completely nervous and silly at this point.

I gave her my phone number and she immediately called me. I could not believe it! I was actually speaking with the person that I almost instantly fell in love with 45 minutes prior online. It turns out that she was from Singapore, is very beautiful, worked in sales in the IT industry, and cooks very good. Long story short, we had a lot in common. We both were looking for someone serious to marry. No games, no dramas. We talked on the phone for 3 hours the first night. Everyday after that we spoke at least 2 to 4 hours per day and chatted online using AOL IM.

Within one month, I had purchased her a round-trip ticket. She flew over from Singapore on August 15, 2000, within a week, we both decided she was going to stay and that we were meant for each other and wanted to stay together and get married. On September 16, 2000 we go married. We definitely rushed into things and once she was here, it seemed everything happened so fast. The reasons that it worked out for us is because:

1. We were very serious about finding someone to marry and spend the rest of our lives with.

2. I was more than two years out of divorce, had dated around and was ready to settle down.

3. She was more than a year out of a four-year relationship and was ready to settle down.

4. We were both very mature, smart individuals that knew exactly what we wanted.

5. We have a lot in common even though we are from different nationalities.

6. We were both ready to make a commitment to each other.

So when you feel you are absolutely ready to give up your status as a single individual and you know for certain that you are ready to make a serious commitment to either a long-term relationship or marriage, develop your plan of action and play the numbers game. In so doing, just remember that there is such a thing as Karma. That is, whatever you cast out into the world will come back to you in like kind. Hence, if you are not serious and end up breaking someone else's heart or hurting their feelings because you are just playing to see what happens, you may end up getting hurt yourself when you are ready to settle down and be serious. Just be careful about how you make your approach and be certain to keep your communication open and honest.

Chapter 45:

"T.E.A.M."

T.E.A.M. – This is both a concept and a lesson. T.E.A.M. stands for Together Everyone Achieves More. This implies that when involved in a group, everyone can get more accomplished by pulling together and acting as a TEAM. You see teams everyday playing football, basketball, soccer and so on. By watching carefully you notice that every member on the team does everything they can to help out to the other members be successful because they too understand this concept. The real lesson to be learned here is that it is not just important for you as an individual to win, rather it is more important that you win as a team. That way everybody wins.

To be on a winning T.E.A.M., you must be coach-able. To be coach-able, you must have a good attitude and be willing to listen and learn. Hence, if you have a good attitude, and are willing to listen and learn, then you are coach-able. It is important to be coach-able because we are working as a team here. I am giving you a lot of lessons and instructions in this book and you must have a good attitude and be willing to listen and learn. Apart from that, you must be willing to apply what you are learning in this book and continue applying it until you have mastered it. That is exactly what professional athletes do in their off season. They continue to practice over and over simple and basic skills until they have mastered them.

So you must practice these important relationship lessons until you have mastered them enough that it comes natural for you. Point being: do not give up if you feel awkward or uncomfortable at first or get knocked down. Continue getting back up and make the conscious effort to do even better the next time while learning from your mistakes. This is how every human being learns new things from the time they are born. This concept works for everyone else and has for thousands of years so do not try to short cut or change it. Embrace it! It works and it will work for you.

Another important thing to remember in being part of a team is that you must be adaptable to new ideas and changing environments. It has been proven that those who are willing to adapt to new and changing environments will succeed and become stronger. I know a lot of people that are very comfortable with where they are and do not take change very well. The fact of the matter is that the only thing you can count on not changing in your life is that fact that everything is going to continue to change. Since everything is going to continue to change in our lives, no matter what we do, why not embrace this fact?

Need some motivation for embracing change? Take a look back at the last five years of your life. If you do not make a change or do something different, the next five years are going to be just like the last five years. I may not know about you but I definitely want to embrace change and continue moving forward!

So how can you apply this TEAM concept to your relationships? Well, the first thing you could use this concept for is going out on double dates. If you have never had the opportunity to go out on a double date, trust me, it is a blast. Simply you along with your date and another couple go out for dinner, a movie, etc. What makes this approach really nice is that the person you are asking out will most likely feel more comfortable knowing that there will be other people around which should put them more at ease and willing to say "Yes". Especially if it is a female, knowing that there will be another female that she can talk to and get to know. Remember, on your first date, you want to take things very slowly and the whole idea is to get to know each other a little better and decide to either continue or not continue dating each other.

Double dating is perfect for this because it gives each of you the opportunity to observe each other while at the same time having another couple with you to help keep the evening and conversation flowing. This way you do not look like an idiot because you either ran out of things to say, have a loss of ideas to suggest, or just plain nervous. Besides, it makes it lot easier on you to ask someone out for a date the first time by being able to ask..."John and Sue are going out for dinner and a movie on Saturday, they invited me to come along with them and I was wondering if you would like to join me?", rather than asking..."Would you like to go out for dinner and a movie on Saturday night?"

Notice the difference? You are more likely to get a "Yes" with the first approach. This is how you use the TEAM approach when it comes to dating. Besides, John and Sue will have a great time as well because it also gives them a chance to see things from a new perspective and meet someone new. As long as the evening goes well without incident, you win! Remember that small commitments lead to larger commitments. You just got past your first small commitment and have paved the road for the next larger commitment, whether it is going out on a date with just the two of you this time, or just going out on a second date period.

Once you have met your ideal mate and gotten past the initial stages of dating and getting to know each other, the TEAM concept continues working in your relationship for either better or worse. I say this because you and your date will eventually see each other as an asset to each other or as a detriment to each other. If you operate and function as a team and each person benefits, this help strengthen the relationship and you will both see each other as an asset and want to continue the relationship. Conversely, if you do not function as a team and it puts a strain on the relationship, eventually the relationship will dissolve. It is up to you to understand this, be adaptable to your new environment and learn to identify ways that this TEAM concept will help strengthen the relationship.

For example: Perhaps your date does not have a washing machine and has to go to a laundry mat to wash clothes, and you do have a washing machine. Invite your date over to do their laundry at your place. Your date wins because this helps them save money and puts them in a more secure environment. You win because you get to spend more quality time with your date, they are in a more secure environment, and you keep them from encountering someone else in the laundry mat that may try to put a move on them or ask them out.

These are just several examples of how the TEAM concept works in relationships. Ultimately, it is up to you to be creative and discover new and exciting ways to make this work so that Together Each of you Achieve More.

Chapter 46:

"Not At This Time"

Not At This Time - I learned this phrase from a networking group I used to belong to. Since learning it, I must have used this phrase at least a thousand times and had great results every time. Here is why. Telling someone "Not At This Time" is a very subtle way of telling someone "No" or "I am not interested right now" without hurting anyone's feelings. You can use this phrase in almost every situation or any occasion. The next time you need to tell someone "No", use the phrase "Not At This Time" instead. Psychologically it makes you feel better about saying "No" and it makes the other person understand that you are saying "No" without hurting their feelings. Hence, psychologically they feel better.

I remember one of the first times that I used this phrase and it worked very well for me. I was in the city walking down the street and on the corner was a man asking everybody that walked by for money. He began arguing and giving everyone that said "No" a hard time. When I approached him, he looked at me and of course, he had to also ask me for money. Little did he know, I was struggling financially too at the time, so I looked back at him square in the eyes and with sincerity said to him, "Not At This Time", in return, he said "OK, thank you sir". I could not believe it. It actually worked and he did not scold me like he did everyone else. I felt good about saying "No" to him in my new found way, and I did not make him feel bad about it, and he actually thanked me instead of giving me a hard time.

What I instantly realized about using this phrase is that psychologically I never actually said "No" to the man. I put myself in his shoes for a moment and thought about what was just said. From his perspective, he understood me to say "not right now, but possibly later". If I ever see him again and he asks me for money again, I'll just tell him "not at this time" again.

This phrase can be used when you are being pressured to purchase something, go out on a date, do something against your will, give an answer, or just about any situation that would make you feel uncomfortable. In most cases it puts the other person at ease and stops them from pressuring you. Keep in mind though, in their minds, they heard you saying "not right now". If nothing else, this will at least buy you some time. So the next time you are being pressured or put in an uncomfortable situation and have to give a response, use the phrase "Not at this time", to either get you out the uncomfortable situation or buy yourself some time.

Chapter 47:

How To Say NO While Saying YES – Sometimes "NO" is not an option because you may hurt someone's feelings, come across as being weak, or place yourself in a difficult situation. In cases like this you will have to understand how to say "NO" while verbally saying "YES". I know this may sound a bit confusing at first and once you understand and learn how to use this concept, you too will become a master at telling people "Yes" and they will clearly understand that you mean "NO".

In order to understand and master this concept, you must first realize that there is a hidden psychological law that most people are not aware of called the "Law of Psychological Reciprocity". The Law of Psychological Reciprocity states that if you give people credit for their intelligence first, then they are morally and subconsciously bound to give you credit for the next thing you say. This also applies when giving physical items or gifts to someone. That is an individual feels compelled to give something back to the person in return for receiving something. Conversely, you are morally and subconsciously entitled to ask for something in return when asked for something. Hence, when someone asks you to give a donation, you are entitled to get back a tax-deduction, small gift or token in return or something.

This sounds all good and well but how do you say NO while saying YES? Very simple, since you are morally and subconsciously entitled to ask for something in return when asked for something, and there are no limitations to what you may ask for in return, why not ask for something that you know the other person will not give or is willing to offer? The way you do this is by answering the person with "Yes, I will do that for you, if you will do _____ for me." Fill in the blank! For example: You ask me to help you move into your new house on Saturday. It just so happens that I already have tickets to a football game that I have been dieing to go see.

Rather than telling you "NO", I could reply back with saying "YES, I will help you move on Saturday, if you will help me paint my entire house on Sunday or make it on Friday, the day before they have to move. Now I already know that you are not going to be willing to help me paint my entire house just for helping you move, however, I did tell you "YES". Now of course you want to use this approach only when you have to.

Another example that I actually used was when I received a telephone call soliciting me for a donation. I have no idea who this person was or if they were legitimate. The way I handled it was by telling the caller..."yes, I would be happy to make a donation if you will first mail me the information on your organization." I already knew that they are not going to do this, so the caller immediately hangs up on me without even saying goodbye. Now obviously if they are going to just hang up on me without even saying "thank you", "goodbye", or "go to hell", then I must have made the right decision of telling the NO while saying YES.

The whole idea is to put the person asking you for something in a position that forces them to give you something of great value in return or to simply back away from asking you for something. This response works every time and you never have to say "NO". Be prepared though, because some people may be willing to give you what you want in return for what they are asking for.

Another way you can use this response is to ask for something that you really do want or need and know that it is very likely the other person may just be willing to give it to you. Take some time to think through how you can use this response and start having fun telling people "NO while saying YES".

Chapter 48:

"There Are Three Sides To Every Story"

There Are Three Sides To Every Story – I had to learn this lesson the hard way. I was always quick to jump to conclusions and take sides whenever my friends would get into an argument with their date or spouse. Of course I would always take the side of the friend I liked the most. It never really occurred to me what I was doing until this started happening with my wife and I. Whenever we would have an argument and need some space or time apart, she would call on some of our friends and go visit them and explain her side of the argument. Doing the same thing that I used to do, they would immediately take her side and I would always look like the bad guy. After a while, this started to infuriate me because they did not even hear my side of the story. Everyone knows when you are upset, you tend to exaggerate details and stretch the truth a little.

You know...five minutes gets exaggerated into thirty minutes or ten dollars gets exaggerated into fifty dollars. This is when I began to learn that there really are three sides to every story. There is your version, the other person's version and then there is the truth somewhere in the middle. My wife and I are still together and will be celebrating our 10th Wedding Anniversary on September 16th 2010. However, as a result of this valuable lesson there are some friends that we no longer hang out or associate with. What ended up happening as a result of our friends not realizing that there were three sides to every story and always taking her side, they began telling my wife that she should leave me and that I was not good enough for her?

Knowing that they only heard her version of what really happened and realizing that she had exaggerated the truth a little, she would never listen to their advice because she knew that was not the right answer to our problems, nor was it the right thing to do. As a result, my wife decided on her own that she no longer wanted to hang around certain friends of ours because all they wanted to do was try to break us up. The sad truth is that had they understood this simple lesson, we would all still be friends.

The important lesson for you to learn here is that whenever someone comes to you and needs to let off some steam because of an argument or disagreement, remember, do not immediately take sides. This only helps fuel the fire. Remember that there are three sides to every story. By not following this rule, you are setting yourself up to lose the friendship of friends and family members. Likewise, when it is you that is involved in the argument, after you have let off your steam, remember to TAKE RESPONSIBILITY and tell the person you are venting to, please do not take sides with me because this is my side of the story and we all know that there are three other sides that they need to know about before forming an opinion or conclusion.

By handling the situation this way, they will bare in mind that you just need to vent off some steam and will continue to support you and not take sides or advise you to take drastic measures. Remember the lesson about Responsibility? It is ultimately up to you to make sure that everyone you speak to completely understands what you are saying and what you mean by what you are saying.

Chapter 49:

"EGO"

EGO – This is one of the biggest if not the biggest relationship killers that I know of. I have seen so many relationships ruined because of this one three-letter word. Ego is the cause of more fights, arguments, wars, and battles than any other reason. It is unfathomable to even comprehend how many relationships have been ruined, lives lost, and friendships split because of ego. In fact, it is so important to you and all of your relationships for you to understand, that I am going to give you the complete definition of ego.

Ego is:

1. The self, especially as distinct from the world and other selves.
2. In psychoanalysis, the division of the psyche that is conscious, most immediately controls thought and behavior, and is most in touch with external reality.
3. An exaggerated sense of self-importance; conceit.
4. Appropriate pride in oneself; self-esteem.

Most often it is an exaggerated sense of self-importance or pride that causes complications and problems between people. Everyone wants to feel important and wants for everyone else to think that they are important. It is in the process of protecting this feeling of pride or self-importance that most of our problems begin. The problem stems from that fact that as human beings, we become emotionally attached to certain thoughts and feelings and through our attachment, feel that we have to protect these thoughts and feelings at whatever cost. For example an outstanding athlete becomes emotionally attached to their thoughts and feelings that they are an outstanding athlete.

If anyone tries to convince them otherwise or make fun of their self-status, the athlete feels emotionally injured and feels compelled to react in such a way as to protect their self-status and self-importance. This reaction could be through verbal expression, physical expression, or mental facial expression. Either way, the athlete is reacting in such a way so as to protect his self-image that he has chosen to become emotionally attached to. The reality is that it is the athlete's emotional attachment to his own self-image and unwillingness to look past his self-image that causes him to allow himself to feel angered. Ultimately, it is his choice to feel hurt and angered and want to retaliate from a sense of trying to protect his own self-image.

If he would learn to look past his own self-image being hurt, and instead realize and accept that ultimately no matter what anyone else says about him, he is still going to be a great athlete and that no words can physically hurt him, he would not be phased by what someone else says or thinks about him. Likewise, when we find ourselves in a situation whereby someone else has said something which hurts our own self-image or self-importance, we too need to look past our own self-image and realize that the words they are speaking can only hurt us if we choose to let them. Otherwise, these words, gestures, actions, or facial expressions cannot touch us and if they cannot touch us, they cannot hurt us.

Since everyone is guilty of having a big ego, the best thing to do is to learn how to manage your ego. Just as you are in control of your thoughts, you are also in control of your ego. The best way to control your ego is by being consciously aware of it. By being aware of it, you consciously decide how you will react or respond to any given circumstance. Remember, whether you choose to be consciously aware of your ego and keep it in control or choose to let it unconsciously control itself, you still have made a choice. Therefore, it is always best to be consciously aware of your ego and keep it in control.

Here are some problems and solutions to some of the most common ways that ego affects your relationships:

1. Thinking that you are better than someone else. This makes you feel superior and look down on the other person or give little significance to their input. SOLUTION: Humble yourself! Consciously remember that everyone was created equal and that no one is better than anyone else. Remember that every human being has feelings that can easily be hurt. Ask yourself if displaying your ego is being a part of the problem or part of the solution?

2. Thinking that you already know everything. This closes your mind to learning new things that you have not even discovered yet. It makes other people feel like they are wasting their time speaking to you because you never listen. SOLUTION: Humble yourself! Learn to listen attentively whenever someone is speaking to you. Amazingly you will begin to learn new and different things and suddenly other people will want to speak to you more often. Also, by listening attentively, you will almost always learn something new or different.

3. Making fun of other people. This may temporarily help your ego but it does nothing to help out a cause. People that are always judging and making fun of other people are insecure and are constantly worried about what other people think about them. SOLUTION: Humble yourself! If you have concerns about your own image, except it and deal with it, almost everyone has some concern about themselves. Learning to accept it and not suppressing it allows you to deal with it and get over it quicker. By learning to make fun of yourself more often, other people will see you as more of a fun person to be around and will not notice your differences as much.

4. Being inflexible or not compromising. Thinking or projecting an image that your way is the only way. Never giving in or allowing someone else to have their way. SOLUTION: Humble yourself! Learn to be flexible. You do not always have to have your way. In a relationship, it is give and take, not take and take. If you want your relationship to be more meaningful and fun, learn to give

in and compromise. Ask yourself, am I doing this for my relationship or am I doing this for just myself? It does not take a rocket scientist to figure out that if you only do things for yourself and not your relationship, eventually your partner is going to leave you.

5. Never admitting that you are wrong or never apologizing. This is a big NO NO! SOLUTION: Humble yourself! Never feel ashamed to admit that you are wrong or apologize for being wrong. It works miracles. Instead of being viewed as an arrogant ass, you will be viewed as someone who is human that admits to making mistakes. I have seen this cause more problems in relationships than any other reason. One partner would not admit to the other that they made a mistake and a large heated argument would ensue. This is the number one cause of frustration in relationships. One person will not admit or apologize for their mistakes and the other person holds grudges. As soon as you realize you made a mistake, apologize for it immediately. Waiting only makes the problem worse.

6. Thinking that you are too good to do something. Thinking you are better than someone else and should not have to perform a certain task, rather they should. SOLUTION: Humble yourself! Never think that you are too good to do something. Never! The moment you do, your partner will become hell bent on leather to get you to do it. It is called reverse psychology. Make them think that you do not want to do something and they will want to make you do it. Make them think that it does not bother you and most likely they will not want to make you do it. Either way, always be willing to help out and do whatever it takes to get the job done and keep the relationship running smooth.

I am sure you can think of occasions when your ego has gotten in your way and when you have seen someone else's ego get in their way. A very important fact for you to remember about being involved in relationships is that very few people will tolerate being involved with someone else having a big ego. You may feel like everything is fine and dandy but believe you me, I learned the hard way with my first wife. I never even suspected it until after the fact. Learn to humble yourself, be consciously aware of your ego and constantly ask yourself everyday, "how can I help, how can I serve", especially when it involves your relationship. Constantly asking these two simple questions will help keep you humble and open your eyes to new opportunities that are right in front of you.

The rule of thumb to remember if ever in doubt is that you can never do too much when it involves helping out your relationship. Most definitely do not take for granted that everything is going to be fine or things will just work themselves out. If there are problems because of an ego, and almost every relationship has them, you had better become aware of them and begin dealing with them one by one. One way or another these problems will be dealt with, either by becoming aware of the ego and correcting the problems or the other person eventually breaking off the relationship.

Chapter 50:

"Emotional Detachment"

Emotional Detachment - If you want to learn to be completely liberated...I mean free-as-a-bird feeling to where nothing can tie you down or hold you back...I mean that wonderful giddy feeling of freedom you get on the first really nice warm day of spring after a long cold winter, then you need to learn to become completely detached emotionally to the outcome of things happening in your life! Remember, it is a choice to decide to be attached or detached to the outcome...the choice is always yours.

The difference however is a feeling of liberation and autonomy or a feeling of being held down by your own concerns to the outcome of something that may or may not ever happen! Just as important as being detached to the outcome is the mental anguish you free up allowing yourself to be even more carefree and creative with your mind, your time, and your decisions. It is amazing how much of your energy and resources you tie up being attached and stuck to the outcome of something.

Being emotionally detached does not mean that you do not care or have concerns; it just means that you have chosen to not let the outcome interfere with the direction you ultimately want to move in or interfere with your emotional psyche or attitude and rob you of your enthusiasm for life. Think about it this way for a moment...a person who is emotionally detached is a lot more enthusiastic and carefree about life than someone who is rigid and stuck in their ways on how something has to end up or play out. Which type of person would you rather be around?

The person who is emotionally attached is usually easily upset, has to have things a certain way, likes to complain a lot, is usually jealous and talks about others, and is usually not very pleasant to be around because their time is so consumed with how something is going to play out or how something has to be done rather than spending their time playing and having fun with the people they are with and letting the universe handle the details for them.

This applies to all of your existing and future relationships because everyone that comes in to contact with you will very quickly determine if you are an emotionally detached and fun person to be with and hang around or are you a rigid and dead set in your ways kind of person. Can you imagine who people like to be around most? Now imagine...who ends up getting more dates, has more friends, and longer-lasting relationships?

So if you have been stuck in your own old ways all of your life, why not take a different approach and have more fun and give yourself permission to be "emotionally detached" to the outcome of whatever it is you are doing? Who knows, this just might free your mind up from anguish long enough for someone to take notice of you smiling and contagious with enthusiasm! And, this is the real hidden secret to why so many people call me smiley. I have had people tell me they saw me driving down the road smiling from ear to ear and I was the only one in the car!

I learned how valuable this lesson is in life and how we can take control of our emotions and chose to be happy and carefree simply by choosing to be emotionally detached to the outcome of whatever it is in our life that tries to rob us of our time, attention and enthusiasm for life!

Chapter 51:

"Embrace Uncertainty"

Embrace Uncertainty - This goes hand-in-hand with being "emotionally detached"! Almost everybody I know is fixated on the outcome of just about everything going on in their life. This means that they are so consumed with the outcome of everything that they have to know how everything is going to turn out and that they are going to be "OK" once everything is said and done.

This is all fine and well except that life does not always work out that way! Sometimes we need to change our ways of doing things instead of doing the same old mundane tasks day after day, week after week, month after month, year after year. Add some excitement and life to your life! I remember when I found the book I mentioned in an earlier chapter titled, "The Seven Spiritual Laws of Success", sitting on my bookshelf...and remember, I was at a point in my life whereby my ex-wife had left me after having an affair, I had a lot of emotional baggage, and honestly the world just sucked for me at that time.

Then one day I walked into my home office and picked up that book titled "The Seven Spiritual Laws of Success" by Deepak Chopra, and this seemed to be the turning point that I needed in my life to pull me past the depression mode I had been in for several months. Up to that moment when I discovered this new book sitting on my bookshelf that I did not recall purchasing nor placing on my bookshelf, I was determined to hold on to everything remaining in my life and wanted it all to remain the same and to not change on me. I was frantically holding on to everything and terrified of anything else changing on me.

This was my safety blanket! As long I knew that everything else in my life would stay the same, I knew eventually I would be alright. This was how I thought I was going to keep my sanity. Then I started reading "The Seven Spiritual Laws of Success" and almost immediately I felt as if this book was written specifically for me because it seemed to address all of the problems and challenges I was facing in life and did not have answers for or know how to deal with. The problems addressed in the book were so realistic and were so accurate to my personal situation that I actually got scared and everything seemed surreal.

It almost felt like somebody was watching me and all of the problems I was going through and had written a book specifically for me. Anyway, one of the very best lessons I learned from Deepak Chopra's book was how to "Embrace Uncertainty". This was absolutely vital for me to learn at this point of my life because everything was flipped upside down, my life was full of unfamiliar feelings and emotions of insecurity and I was an absolute emotional mess trying to grab, claw, and hold on to anything and everything I possibly could that had some sense of familiarity to me.

All I knew was that everything in my life was changing faster than I was emotionally capable of keeping up with and up to that moment, life was very stressful! Then for whatever reason, I discovered and started reading this new book conveniently placed on my bookshelf as if the hand of GOD pulled it out of thin air and set it in front of me...knowing the state of mind I was in and what type of emotional help I needed. Whoever or whatever placed that book there for me to notice and read, THANK YOU!...because it was the turning point of my life that got me back on my feet emotionally and allowed me to pick myself back up again and dust off my shoulders.

Some of the vitally important lessons I learned from reading this one chapter "Embrace Uncertainty" in "The Seven Spiritual Laws of Success" was that life is unpredictable and that we must learn to come to the realization of this. I also learned that by being rigid and determined to what I expected the outcome to be, in whatever situation or circumstance I was in, I was robbing myself of the excitement of the unknown and caused myself a lot more grief and stress than normal.

What I realized was that by letting go of my perception of what I felt had to be the end result of something happening in my life (letting go of having to know what the outcome was going to be), I had a lot less stress to deal with, I was a lot more relaxed and accepting towards myself and everyone else around me. I then realized that for the first time in a long time I was now open for other possibilities that life offers. Because I was not so fixated on the outcome having to be a certain way, I would not miss other opportunities that were presenting themselves to me as well. This freed up even more emotional stress and actually gave me a sense and feeling of freedom and excitement because I now had this new found sense of how to embrace uncertainty, that I knew that whatever the outcome was, I was going to be OK and able to deal with it by embracing even more uncertainty!

Furthermore, I realized that by not knowing what the outcome was going to be with any given situation going on in my life, I was allowing myself to go back to our true human nature. Our true human nature is designed to "embrace uncertainty" because we live in a world of so many possibilities that there simply cannot be one answer that fits or works for everybody all the time.

Therefore, by learning to "embrace uncertainty", we effectively allow ourselves to be open to other possibilities that are more suited for who we are and not stuck with an outdated answer or possibility that may have worked well for someone else but not us. Let others be fixated on the outcome while you vibrantly look forward to life's exciting uncertainties and embrace them. These other possibilities can only surface or materialize if we are open to "embracing uncertainty" and not dead-set on how something has to play out or end up. Think of it as either being a tall old oak tree that is rigid and set in it's way which snaps and breaks when a rough wind blows or being like a reed of grass that is flexible and bendable and adaptable and does not break in half when a rough wind blows.

I decided that I no long wanted to be like the rigid oak trees, set in my own ways, which snaps and breaks in a storm, rather, I wanted to be like the reed of grass that was flexible and adaptable and embraced the uncertainty of the storm and survived. What I also gained from this valuable lesson was how exciting it really is to live life again without having preconceived notions of how everything needed to end up according to my expectations. Rather, I rediscovered the excitement of learning new things for the very first time again in my life because I am now able to embrace uncertainty.

It is comparable to the excitement of being a kid all over again being able to discover new and exciting things for the very first time again! Once you learn to allow yourself (by giving yourself permission) to embrace uncertainty, everyday then becomes an exciting, fun-filled adventure full of excitement and surprises which changes your outlook, which changes you psychosomatically, which changes your outward appearance and energy level which attracts more and exciting people toward you.

So go ahead and let down your guard give yourself permission to embrace uncertainty and when your gut feeling is telling you to do something new and different and exciting and your mind is telling you "No, you have to do it the same old way you have always done it", go with your gut feeling and embrace uncertainty and rediscover what it is like to be excited about life again and all of the uncertainties that it brings with it, day by day! Life really is exciting...if you allow it to be.

Chapter 52

"RESPECT"

RESPECT - One of the most important lessons I learned while growing up as a kid was to show respect towards others. Now, I will be the first to admit that over the years it has been my choice to not always adhere to this policy, but for the most part I genuinely show respect toward other people.

What I have learned about showing respect toward other people is that sometimes you may not see the rewards immediately. Sometimes, it takes years to see the benefit. This makes it that much more challenging to be respectful toward some people especially when they are directly correlated to your feelings, and emotions, and heart being crushed.

Even still we must learn to pull ourselves together and continue pressing forward and be respectful none-the-less. This belief paid off for me one day when I was patching things up with my wife, Rose, when she told me several days after we had an argument that even though we were pretty mad at each other during the argument, and that she purposely said some things to make me feel upset, she told me she admired the fact that I kept my composure and in spite of how mad I was at her, I continued to treat her with respect, and that because I did continue to show her respect, she admired that characteristic in me and wanted to continue moving forward with our relationship.

This one incidence brought me full circle with my own belief and convinced me to continue being respectful to others despite what might be temporarily happening on the outset. That sometimes, people may purposely say or do things to you just to see how you will react. Good, bad, or indifferent, you just have to accept the fact that some people will chose to put you through this test before they will let down their guard and let you in.

And just like the old saying goes, "the game is not over until the clock stops ticking", the same is true with being respectful toward others, "continue being respectful toward others until you are the last person standing". Even if everything ends up going in the wrong direction, you will still be admired by the people around you for remaining respectful.

Sometimes it is not the person that you are being respectful towards that will ultimately make you happy. Sometimes it's the people that are watching you to see how you react that will ultimately end up making you happy because you kept your composure and demonstrated yourself as someone they would like to be with.

So remember, when you get put in an uncomfortable spot in any of your relationships, always keep your composure and remain respectful at all times because you never know who else is watching you or how your decisions may ultimately affect your outcome.

Chapter 53:

"SEX"

SEX - Let's be honest with ourselves on this one. Sex is something that we all love and crave for. It is the end result of what we are ultimately after when we get involved in a romantic relationship and yet is probably the one thing that we will work our absolute hardest and do some of the most craziest things in the world for. Think about it, we will go without food, water, and sleep but we refuse to go without sex. I know I cannot go without it. It helps me to relieve stress, feel pleasures like no other, and brings me intimately close to the person I love the most. Not to mention it helps us procreate babies.

As long as there is sex in our relationship(s), our relationship(s) seem good, right? Well this is where it gets complex, because if most of everything else mentioned in this book is not in proper order, you can pretty much kiss the sex part goodbye. Take it from me personally, because I know first hand how this works. You see as long as I keep my wife in check and follow the advice I mention in my own book, we have great sex. As soon as I start to get off course a little, there goes the sex part out the window, immediately. Sometimes I feel like I'm wearing an invisible collar. As long as I have it on, I am good to go....as soon as I take it off I am in the doghouse again.

Sex is pretty straightforward for men, we like it, we want it, we search out for it and we find it. For women it is a lot more complicated. Most women want to feel loved and appreciated before having sex, and rightfully so. It works kind of like a reward system. If you have romantic feelings towards each other and do what you are supposed to you get to have sex. If you do not have romantic feelings towards each other and do what you are supposed to do or what is expected of you, you do not get to have sex.

All kidding aside though, you should view sex as the glue that helps keep the relationship going through the tough times. It helps you bond, and feel intimate, and close with each other. On the other side, lack of sex can be the cause of cheating, promiscuity, and the breakup of otherwise great relationships. You should consider sex and communication as the top two most important factors for a long term sustained romantic relationship.

It kind of works like a double edged sword, if everything is moving along just fine in your relationship, then your life and relationship are just great! As soon as things start going sideways in your sex life, the relationship part of it starts to crumble, and then you are start to having serious problems in your relationship.

Let me elaborate some for both men and women. Men, respect your lady and do the very best you possibly can to care and support her and make an effort to win her over every single day. Go back to doing some of the things that you did for her when you wanted to win her over. She will eventually become ecstatic and feel obliged and look up to you.

Women, you need to understand some basic simple facts about men and sex. It is the one thing in life we choose not to live without. If you cannot keep your man sexually happy, eventually, he will end up finding that happiness somewhere else. He just may not always tell you about it. Also, do not play games with men when it comes to sex, because eventually they will leave you over someone else that can make them sexually satisfied.

I have seen it happen time and time again. Just like us men have to keep doing our very best we can one day at a time to win over our women, women need to also keep doing the very best they can do one day at a time to help keep the sex life happy, because if the sex life is happy, the man will almost always go out of his way to help you.

Women, if you have never heard this before, please pay close attention to what I am telling you right now. Do Not Play Games With Sex! If you choose to, do not let it be a surprise to you if you get dumped and left all alone because you chose to play games when it came to sex. Men do not like playing games when it comes to sex. We take this very seriously. Now all of this advice about sex is with the understanding that the relationship is at a point whereby you both are ready to begin having sex in your relationship.

So, if you are involved in a new relationship, obviously sex is not something you have to be that concerned about at first. Mind you though, it will become an issue very quickly, and how you approach and deal with it will to a large extent determine the success of your new relationship.

So when it comes to sex, remember men and women take this very seriously and men will go without food, water, and rest to obtain it. Women want to have the feeling of being loved, respected, and cared for, and rightfully so. Above all else, keep in mind that sex is something to be enjoyed by both parties when the timing is right and not something to be used as a mind game or control process, because long-term that never works.

Chapter: 54

"All You Can Do Is All You Can Do"

All You Can Do Is All You Can Do - At some point you may have to come to the realization that you have really and truly done all that you possibly can do to help make the relationship work. Believe it or not there are some rare cases when someone will actually change for the better. They will do this because they really want to change and they are ready to change to make their life better, not because you want them to.

I say it this way because you cannot force someone to change their ways, especially just because you want the change. I was one of those rare individuals that really and truly deep down inside wanted to change and I was ready to change. Nobody could have forced me to change, and up til the point that Rose came into my life, I didn't want to change.

Once you have completely exhausted all possibilities and you know deep down inside that even with all of your effort things are just not going to work out in the relationship, no matter what, it is time to move on with your life and leave the person who is unwilling to change and is holding you back from having the ideal relationship. Otherwise you will just end up being miserable tolerating a relationship that does not bring the full potential out of you.

An idea you can always consider for breaking things off easily is by letting the person know that you have decided to move on with your life because you have made every effort possible (or are willing) to make the relationship work and that for right now it is best for both of you to spend some time apart so that each of you can work on getting your own individual lives back in order and then consider dating each other again afterwards. You want to do this because apparently some things are not working out the way they should.

If the other person is just obsessed with you and will not leave you alone, you definitely know you made the correct decision to break things off. If on the other hand they honestly and truly do work and improve you have some options to consider. The key here is to create as much time and distance between the two you as possible for as long a period of time as possible. The more time that passes, the more the other person has to learn to become independent of you and will either improve or continue spiraling downward.

In the meantime, you continue focusing ahead and continue improving yourself one day at a time, and remember we succeed or fail by our self in 24 hour time blocks. It is YOUR freedom and CHOICE to decide to stay or move on!

Chapter: 55

"NEXT"

NEXT- Next is the next step you take after you have done all you can either possibly or are willing to do to save your relationship and have decided it is time to move on. After you have verbally and expressly set things in motion to let the other person know that things are over between you, you walk outside into the middle of the street and look straight up in to the air and as loud as you can, yell NEXT!!!!

It really does feel great and it gets you over any hang-ups you might be having. So the next time you get involved in a relationship and realize you made the wrong CHOICE, follow you gut instincts and if that involves breaking off the relationship in order to keep your sanity, do so and then run out in to the street and yell it as loud as you can and then make a commitment to move on with your life and do the very best you can do one day at a time.

Chapter: 56

"OK"

"OK" - If there was one word in the entire world that could be directly correlated to making life a lot easier, it would have to be the word "OK". Learn to say "OK" often! OK!? Learning to just shut my mouth and say "OK" has been a blessing in disguise and helped me stay out of more trouble than I would like to admit. All joking aside, learning to use the word "OK" can do volumes towards keeping you in good standing and out of harms way in all of your relationships. Honestly, this one word works with every single one of your relationships...family, business, love, and friends!

For example: I remember watching a TV show that had me enthralled and right as there was a build-up of suspense that I did NOT want to miss, my lovely wife decides it is time to ask if I can help her vacuum the rugs!? At first I sat there and pretended like I did not hear what she said and that worked for about 30 seconds. Then came the second request! I looked over at her and said, let me finish watching my show first.

Apparently that was a big mistake because she started getting louder and louder with her conversation and questions toward me and the next thing you know we were arguing over everything under the sun because I would not get up right then and there to vacuum some rugs that were not going anywhere. Now come to find out she had a very long day working and was tired and had very little patience at that moment.

What I realized was that if I had just said "OK", I'll get to it as soon as the movie is over. She would have been just fine! Nothing else would have been said! There would have been no long winded discussions about things that did not happen or did not exist. She simply would have gone on about her business and I could have enjoyed finish watching the movie. So from now on, the next time she asks me to help her do anything...I simply say "OK" and let her know when I am available to do whatever it is she needs help with.

So when you find yourself in a situation of being torn between doing something you really enjoy doing and are being summoned by someone else to give them your time and / or attention, remember to use the word "OK" let them know when you are available and notice how much easier your life is the rest of that day.

Chapter: 57

"Those That Play Together"

Those That Play Together – Those that play together stay together. Very short, sweet, and simple. It is a proven fact that couples that have fun together finding things of interest in common together, enjoy longer and more prosperous relationships. So if you really want to see your relationship blossom and prosper and be fun and exciting, find things to do in common and have fun doing them. Rose and I love playing tennis and driving to the beach and mountains. Sometimes it's fun to just drive there, hang out for a little bit, do some shopping or have lunch and then drive back.

Every time you do something like this together, you are strengthening your relationship and bond with each other. Choose to find out what the two of you can do together that is fun, exciting, and involves both of you and go do it no matter what. Just get started and you will see how much fun you will start to have. You don't have to wait for the perfect weather, or perfect weekend or day...just get up and go! Make it spontaneous and carefree sometimes and watch how much fun it is and how strong your bond becomes.

When you go to the park, bring a Frisbee or football. The key is to be active together and play together and have fun together. So in order to make your relationship more fun, exciting, and adventurous, find some things that the two of you can do together, even if it is just the two of you, commit to having fun together and enjoy strengthening your relationship bond.

Chapter: 58

"Get An Animal Together"

Get An Animal Together - getting an animal together gives you something in common to care about and take care of. More importantly, this having an animal takes a lot of the attention off each other, which helps reduce tension between each other, and provides a pathway for the two to begin their relationship together.

It also gives you something to look forward to throughout the day and sets the stage for the responsibility of having kids. Almost every couple I know of had an animal before they had any children, Rose and myself included, so there must be something to it.

It was actually funny, because Rose came from Singapore and did not have any animals while she was growing up and within the first 5 months of use being together, we obtained our dog Cindy and our cat Mooshi. Then one day I came home from work and she had our other dog Sweetie sitting on her desk in our home office just laying back like she had already owned the place.

I immediately asked Rose, why Sweetie was in our house and not across the street at our neighbors (who supposedly owned Sweetie). Rose said the we now own Sweetie because she could not stand to see Sweetie sit outside on the neighbors porch in 19 degree weather freezing. So she walked over to our neighbors house, asked her is she was not going to take of Sweetie, if we could have her and provide her a nice home? Our neighbor, told Rose that she had been waiting for somebody to come by and take Sweetie away from there and would love for Rose to have her.

As soon as Rose told me about Sweetie, I immediately felt sorry for her and knew that we could not get rid of her, even though that was my first reaction. I knew right then that Rose had a soft heart for animals and would most likely have the same maternal concerns for her baby should she ever have one. Well of course we did and even though I had the same knee jerk reaction as I did with Sweetie, I remembered that Rose has a loving and caring heart and after a few days, I came around to the fact of us having a baby together. My life has never been happier since!

We now have our three dogs and one cat and one daughter and everyday is completely filled with love and joy and laughter. So the next time you are wondering what you can do to add some spice to your relationship and help bring out the best in both of you, consider getting an animal together.

Chapter: 59

"Be Pleasantly Persistent"

Be Pleasantly Persistent - We all know that in order to succeed in life you must be Persistent. Just like when you were a baby, you could not walk at first, and then you became persistent and continued being persistent until you started walking. Well the same persistence is required for finding, maintaining, and improving your relationships.

In order to find the right person, you must be very persistent because it becomes a very involved process. Sometimes very similar to a game of cat and mouse because you are dealing with someone you know absolutely nothing about, who has opened themselves up to the rest of the world and you care competing against other people you cannot see, talk to or know anything about. It is like trying to hit a moving target while being blind folded. So persistence is a definite must!

Now let us pretend that you found the perfect person or you feel like you are currently involved in what could become the perfect relationship, now you have to figure out how to maintain the relationship. This means keeping things on an even keel and keeping the relationship interesting by constantly doing things they do not become mundane or boring after the first three times of them. So again persistence is needed to continually be on the ball to keep things going in the right direction.

Now let us pretend that you have found the perfect person to be involved with, you have mastered maintaining the relationship and now you want to improve on certain areas of the relationship to get it to the ideal status that you are looking for. Here again persistence is needed because you may be involved in learning some new habits, activities, or adventures that will help move the relationship in a better direction.

For example, let's say that you are happy with the status of your relationship and feel that it definitely has room for improvement. Knowing that rule of "Those That Play Together Stay Together", you could CHOOSE to introduce some new activities to your relationship that will work towards strengthening and building your relationship bond. Again this can include tennis, golf, racquet ball, volley ball, basketball, bowling...pretty much anything that involves physical activity.

So sometimes the other person may not feel as optimistic as you and you have to continue to be persistent to get them up and going... knowing that once they get involved in the activity, they will have fun and end up enjoying them self and the time spent with you while unknowingly to them helping to build your relationship stronger the entire time.

So when you feel your relationship needs a little push and you feel like the only one pushing, be persistent and realize that once you get to a certain point being involved in the activity you are pushing for, the other person will begin having fun and be thankful that you persistence pushed them to step outside of the comfort zone and not allowing them to just settle. I once heard someone famous say that settling is ok for chickens or cows or sheep but not for humans.

We must constantly keep evolving to feel good about ourselves and each other, and the only way to keep a relationship evolving is through activity and the only way to be active is through persistence. So be persistent and keep on pushing to make your relationships better.

Chapter: 60

Psychological Reciprocity - Psychological Reciprocity is an unwritten rule dealing with human psychology that states that when someone pays you a compliment or makes a compelling statement to you, you are psychologically bound to return a compliment or compelling statement in return, whether good or bad. For example, is someone tells you that you look great and you have a beautiful family, because of your human nature, you are psychologically bound to return a similar type of positive compliment.

As long as this unwritten rule stays in balance, the relationship will maintain enough stability to prosper. If things become unbalance, meaning you begin to notice that you give compliments and they are not reciprocated back to you, eventually you will become concerned about the stability of the relationship because you will feel the other person in the relationship is not reciprocating back to you psychologically, and subconsciously will cause you to start to become concerned about the relationship and it's stability.

This is important to understand for all relationships that you have in your life, whether they be someone you want to have an affair with, marry, or someone in your family because we all have this expected reciprocating psychological response programmed in to us. Therefore, we expect it without having to tell you. We also know that if the reciprocating response is not present in the relationship, it is a clear indication that one person is not as interested in the relationship as the other.

We can sense this before the other person ever says a word to us. You may recall being involved in a relationship and you had this feeling like something was not right or the other person was going to end up breaking things off and you started becoming concerned about. Well that feeling stems from exactly what we are talking about right now.

So as you begin to think through all of your relationships, including any new ones, remember to think carefully how psychological reciprocity can serve as a barometer for the health of your relationships. Take close notice to the responses you get when you give compliments and that should be an indicator to you for their level of strength.

If you receive genuine compliments back when you give them, this indicates that the relationship is strong, if on the other hand the response is weak, then you should quickly realize that this relationship needs some close attention and further observation if you want the relationship to be successful.

Chapter: 61

"Pick-up Lines"

Pick-up Lines – here are some proven and effective pick-up lines to use to ask others out on a date or dinner. These are designed to work for both men and women.

In Person:
Hi, my name is _____, I could not help myself from noticing how very attractive you look today / or how bright your smile is today / or how energetic you are today / or how great you smell today. Please forgive me, I am a little nervous right now and I realize that we do not know each other...so I wanted to take this opportunity to find out if it would possible for the two of us take some time to have some coffee, or tea, or dinner if you feel up to it, so we can have a chance to spend some time getting to know each other?

If YES: That sounds great, how does your schedule look over the next two days? Be careful not to be too anxious. Be calm and relaxed and confident and do not talk too much. If it is not possible to meet up right then and there and you have to schedule for up to two days out, the best thing you can do is get the commitment, let the person you just met know that you are so happy to have met them, and that you are looking forward to meeting up with them on the date and time the two of you specified. After this, let them know that you have to be going and to please enjoy the rest of their day!

You want to get out of there as quickly as you reasonably can simply because while being in a state of nervousness, you may begin babbling and saying things that may cause concern on the other person's part. By leaving, you have time to carefully think through how you want things to flow and can practice what you would like to say to start the relationship off on the right foot. Besides, the other person may be just as nervous and may need to some time as well.

If NO: Well it was nice having the opportunity to briefly speak with you, maybe I will see you around some time. Always leave a positive impression and remember persistence. Just because they said "NO" this time, does not mean "NO" forever. They may have been caught off guard and that was they're first initial response. There could be a million reasons why they said "NO" and you may never know why until later on after you have a chance to get together and they tell you why they said "NO"

The other bold alternative you can use is to challenge their response by saying "obviously you have a reason for saying that, do you mind if I ask what it is?" You want to do this especially if you keep getting told "NO" almost all of the time to figure out what it is that is causing people to say "NO" to you. Unless you ask, they will not voluntarily tell you. At the same time you need to be able to handle some constructive criticism.

Online Internet Profile / Email:
Hi, I could not help myself from noticing your profile and how attractive you look in your photo. I would like to arrange for the two of us to meet up for some coffee, tea, or dinner to have a chance to get to know each other. I know you are probably inundated with replies from other people so please get back with me at your earliest convenience. I really look forward to your reply. You want to add in this little bit of humor towards the end so the other person does not feel so stuffy and gets the sense that they can relax and just be themselves with you.

The email I used to attract Rose goes something like this. "Hello _____(online profile name). I could not help but notice your profile on _____(name of website). Your beauty is what caught my eye, but your love is what will keep me. If you are still in search of someone who is serious about a fun and fulfilling relationship and knows how to treat a lady, please reply back and let me know so we can begin getting to know each other and see if there are sparks between us.

Please keep in mind that I sent this same email out to 25 women all at the same time not knowing who would respond or how many responses I would get. Even though I received 15 replies back, it was Rose that I was most interested in hearing from and heard back from first. It's weird because when I first saw her online profile, my heart starting racing, my face was blushing and my palms started sweating. This all happened before I even emailed her or talked to her.

I knew almost instantly that Rose was the one I wanted to be with and that I could not just sit back in hopes of one person out of millions to respond back to me with mutual feelings. So as I said, my email was sent out to 25 women living in various parts of Asia. All along though my heart was aching and my mind racing with thoughts until Rose responded back to me. Fortunately she was the first person to reply back within about an hour and what seemed like eternity to me.

As soon as she replied back, she asked me for my phone number and immediately called me and from the first day onward, we talked for about 4 hours on the phone. We both knew what we were looking for and just had to be patient and persistent long enough until we found each other. The rest is history and that is how this book was inspired.

So the next time you set out to meet someone new to bring in to your life, remember how important the "Lines" you use are and the impact they can have on the rest of you life just as they have with mine.

Chapter: 62

"Good Morning"

Good Morning – Our attitude and outlook on our entire day is formed within the first five minutes we wake up. Therefore, it is vitally important to your personal and professional success to CHOOSE to start your day off in the right frame of mind and continue reminding yourself throughout the day to keep your attitude and outlook in check.

I personally do this with a simple mantra at the start of each day. This helps me start my day off with a great attitude and lasts throughout the entire day. As a result, I have a lot more successes than failures simply because I expect to succeed. My mantra is very simple and easy to remember..."I am grateful and I expect to succeed".

I am grateful for everything I have up to this point in my life and I expect to continue succeeding. This starts my day off with gratitude for everything I have around me and the expectancy that I will succeed throughout my day. To carry this even further, I constantly ask myself, "how can I help and how can I serve?"

This also helps keep my ego in check and helps me focus on what I can do to help those in need around me and remain humble and as a result success is inevitable.

Chapter: 63

"Stars"

Stars – Did you realize that every one of us is made out of a star? Broken down to our most essential elements every part of us exists only because of the light and warmth we receive from the Sun. Take away the light from the Sun and we all die. The sun gives us Vitamin D for our bones, Chlorophyll for our plants which gives us life, and warmth to keep the Earth from freezing over. Every living human, creature, organism, and plant has sustained life as a result of the Sun. And what is the Sun? It is a Star. Since all of us are all made up of Starlight and have sustained life as a result of this starlight, never lose sight of the fact that you too are a star.

Clearly this emphasizes the importance of every living thing on Earth. When closely examined, we all live in a fragile fabric of co-existence. As a result, everyone should take full advantage of every opportunity they are given. Reach out and claim what can rightfully be yours in this short span of time you are privileged to be here. If starlight can reach out billions of miles to give you sustained life, certainly you can reach out and take full advantage of every opportunity you are given to claim what can be rightfully yours. No one has more privilege over anyone else when it comes to taking full advantage of your opportunities. Some people may want you to believe that they are more privileged and have more right than you, and yet it is up to you to realize and understand that they do not. Remember, God created everyone equally and gave us starlight to help sustain our lives.

Above all else, never ever sell yourself short or look down on yourself because you too are just as much a shining star as everyone else no matter what problems or misfortunes you may seem to have in your life. If the truth were really to be known, we would all realize that all of us have personal problems and issues no matter how attractive they may look or how well they present themselves. Some people are just better at covering up their problems than others. In fact these are the people that you really want to be cautious about because by trying to disguise or cover up their problems, they are not being true to themselves and everyone else around them.

So the next time you are faced with a challenging decision to speak to someone or ask someone out, or stand up for what you believe in, or feel is rightfully yours, remember, we are all made up of the same starlight and that no person is made up of better elements than another. Also, remember to respect the fact that every person has their own personal problems, and you may not always know about them.

Chapter : 64

"Effective Email Tactics"

Ever wondered why you did not get a reply back to your email? Maybe your message was way too dull or deep. An engaging email banter with a potential date can be downright tantalizing. Follow these tips for crafting lively emails to increase your chances of getting a potential date's attention:

1. Cyber Dating 101

Did you spell the person's name correctly? While this would seem to be a given, always use spell check or at least re-read your email to make sure your spelling is correct. Misspelled words are one of the first big turn-offs and silently says a lot about your level of intelligence. The overuse of explanation points or other punctuation marks might make someone wonder about the I.Q. of the sender or their level of sophistication. Avoid it!!!

2. Ask About Interests & Qualities

Ditch the canned, form letter responses that focus on you. Turn it on the other person. People love to talk about themselves, remember the radio station "WIIFM" (What's In It For Me). Engage your potential partner(s) by asking about their favorite hobbies, sports, pets or other interest mentioned in their online ad or posting. Invite detailed feedback on qualities they seek in a potential love affair by asking them more about their ad. This shows that you actually read their ad and are genuinely interested in learning more about them versus just making a quick judgment based on their photo.

3. Charm Still Matters
Remember your manners and be observant, this goes a long way online. Answering questions and keeping your responses in line with the flow of the email will always work better in your favor. Blowing off an appropriate question or being a pushy braggart that just wants to close the deal or talk about themselves are big turnoffs.

4. Trust Your Gut
After just a few online exchanges with someone you will usually get a sense from the content and style of their emails about what makes them tick. Based on what you have learned and experienced up to this point in your life, use your gut instinct to help determine if this is going in the right direction for you and your safety. Use the old "give them enough rope to hang themselves" method. Encourage them to open up some and notice how their focus is affected. You will find clues aplenty: From all-about-me types (embellish in and about themselves), status seekers (I drive a Benz, baby), idealistic humanitarians (Save the Whales volunteer) to the flakier-than-a-piecrust type (look for unanswered questions, short attention spans). Trust your gut instinct on this one.

5. Think Quickly
What would Jim Carey do? He'd improvise and word associate. If you aren't blessed with a quick wit, throw in a short clean joke you've heard recently, state the common uncommonly. Whether you're a movie buff, romantic at heart or avid reader, try quoting some favorite lines that are universal enough to be recognized. ("Somebody stop me" or "You talkin' to me?")

6. Avoid Email Slang
IMHO (In my humble opinion) tread lightly, WRT (with respect to) "emoticons," you know those symbols and acronyms used in emails. Most of the online scene knows that :-) denotes a smile, but a recipient may not know %-) means the sender is confused or that ROTFL finds them rolling on the floor laughing. All this can come in to play later after you have established yourself and feel comfortable with each others expecations.

7. Keep It Clean
Today's electronic chat boards can be no different than bathroom walls. While it might go without saying that rude comments and

obscene come-ons are a definite no-no for most of the masses, a surprising number of women still report receiving emails of this nature. The newbies and even experienced online visitors might be lured by coy emails in initial communications with a potential date, only to be instantly propositioned once they engage in a live online chat. Be courteous – be clean.

Chapter : 65

"Online Dating Tips 101"

I have corresponded with many of my friends about how I was so successful in finding and attracting my wife. After spending some time thinking about it for a few days, I realized the importance of the steps I outlined for myself and came up with the following "10 Online Dating Tips" to help keep your online profile from just sitting there like a boring lump on a log, hardly drawing attention.

It's not hard to create a profile that not only attracts more attention but produces more responses. It just takes a bit of creativity and inspiration. Do these 10 things to get started you started down the right path:

1. Create A Unique & Catchy Headline
Like the front page of a newspaper or magazine draws your eyes to a story, a great headline can draw eyes to your profile. Use it to say something distinctive, as well as highlight your best attributes: The one I used to attract Rose was "Your Beauty is what will attract me, Your Love is what will keep me". You can also use something like "In shape and looking for Match to set the East Coast on fire". Be creative and exciting and add in some humor.

2. Don't Oversell Yourself
Remember, that your online profile is not a resume to become a Rocket Scientist. Be selective with how you describe your best features. For example, "attractive" is a relatively safe way to imply you're comfortable and confident with the way you look. "Very good looking" or "Gorgeous" or "Strikingly handsome" or "Bombshell"

just makes you sound like you are conceited and stuck on yourself. Other alternatives are to talk about the fact that you are an "avid reader," "animal lover" or "family person".

3. Choose A Photo That Compliments You
Sure, you thought that picture of you in the floppy hat at the beach made you look as cute as a button. But since you're trying to attract dates — not your mother, shoot for something a bit more mature and flattering. Remember to avoid photo that shows you being embraced, squeezed or otherwise involved with another person. Don't make it look like you're already taken.

4. Avoid Mentioning the "EX"
No one wants to hear about how you're looking for someone to help you lick your wounds and get over the person who plucked out your heart and stomped it into the gutter of despair. Let it go.

5. List Your Favorite Things
We all would like to climb Mount Everest or sail the globe, but let's be realistic — how many times in a lifetime does that happen? Instead, highlight your ritual weekend bicycle ride or your collection of 70s classic rock. You probably shouldn't mention your collection of 70s classic pornography.

6. Be Reasonable
Limit your list to maybe five favorite things or so. Otherwise, potential matches will think you're just too much into yourself. And, besides, you will want to save something to talk about on your first dates.

7. Keep It Intriguing and Interesting
How many potential matches truly want to join you while you "hang out with the guys" or search for the best beer prices? Instead, describe your more inspired goals.

8. Use Spell Check
Remember, your profile is a reflection of your personality. Misspelled words, poor grammar and too many clichés can be big turnoffs to potential dates. I find that actually printing it out and proof-reading whatever I write helps me catch more errors than by just reading it

on the computer monitor. So consider printing it out first just to be certain it is ready to be sent.

9. Don't Be Too Demanding
Don't say you're looking for the "perfect match with the perfect body." They don't exist, and saying that what you want looks you're above everyone else.

10. Lighten Up and Have Fun
Your free profile should not only be informative but entertaining. Keep it light, engaging and refreshing.

Chapter 66

"How To Go From "Dull" To "Daring"

When it comes to dating, people spend a lot of time preparing themselves so they'll make a good impression. But just as important as looking good is having a well-thought-out plan or theme for the date itself. Taking in a movie, or going to a restaurant — these are the ordinary date activities that can quickly grow dull.

When a date becomes "ordinary," it makes you look plain, unremarkable — and boring. So how do you make your time with that special person stand out? How do you break out of the cookie-cutter mold of an "ordinary date" and give your partner a unique memory that makes you center stage? Here are a few effective suggestions that I have learned from some dating pros.

1. Throw Party For Two:
Jill and I had gone out a few times and since she had invited me to her place, I wanted to reciprocate. She might have been expecting a typical "guys place" with dirty clothes and pizza boxes on the floor, but when she saw my Hawaiian shirt, and the pineapple drink I handed to her as she came in, plus the lei I placed around her neck, she knew she was in for a treat. The theme was 'Hawaiian Luau,' and even though it was the dead of winter, and there was no beach or roasting pig on a spit, Jill got right into the spirit of things and even did a hula dance for me later on. The whole thing took less than a half hour to prepare (plus about an hour to do the shopping). It really made the evening special.

2. Mix Up A Casual Event:

Most of the girls I know have never ridden in a limousine, other than when they went to their high school prom. I was going to pick Stephanie up, and we were just going to hang out at a local coffee house for the afternoon and have lattes and read through the "For Sale" items in the newspaper. You can only imagine her surprised look when she opened the door and saw the limo — her eyes lit up and the biggest smile you ever saw was on her face. The whole time we sat drinking coffees — while the limo and driver waited parked up the street — she just kept giggling and smiling. Then we had a leisurely drive through the streets before taking her home. She had a great time and so did I. (By the way, I do have a car. I just thought the limo would be more fun and make our date stand out. And I was right.)

3. Find A Logical "Next Step"

I like normal dates like going to movies and eating out, but I try to make things more memorable. So I look for a continuing thread to what we're doing. For example, after we saw one of Sean Connery's movies, my date and I went to a bookstore to check out other things written by the director and author. On another occasion, while having a drink in a restaurant, I pointed out the intricate designs on the dining room's molding, and we ended up getting a fascinating mini-discourse on the history of the building from the owner. These types of things "extend" the date and make it much more interesting and memorable.

4. Go Looking For A Thrill

While it's not something you can do on a first date, I have found that when a girl is willing to try something unusual and "scary", it means she's got the kind of spunk that I find appealing. Cynthia and I hit it off from the very beginning, and we went hot air ballooning on our second date. It was not only fun, but also something that we still talked years later. I can only imagine that now she's trying to figure out who she can get to take her hang gliding.

Chapter 67

"Gift Giving Rules"

I can't speak much for anyone else. I do know for sure that as far as I can remember, I always gave gifts. After marrying my wife Rose, she told me a story about a guy she once dated who strategically picked fights with her right before some of the major holidays — Christmas, her birthday, Valentine's Day, especially since her birthday and Valentine's Day are so close together. By the time Valentine's Day had passed, she said she had pretty much gotten the picture.

As she sat alone one day thinking things through, she realized that it shouldn't be this hard. Guys should not have to freak out at the thought of buying a gift for the special person in their lives. So fellows listen up; She said what you need is a simple formula to follow so that you do not end up giving a set of cup holders to your future wife or worse, diamonds to a dame doomed to be a one-night stand. So after some serious thought, and talking to some friends of ours, Rose and I came up with this simple formula for gift giving.

Gift Giving 101
When considering buying gifts for someone you are dating, you need to consider a few things first:
How long have you been dating?
How long do you want to continue dating?

Applying The Rules
Make no mistake about it, the upcoming holidays can add a whole new set of pressures to dating and gift-giving. So take some of the pressure off of yourselves and apply the same gift-giving formula

and think about the message you want to send about the future of your relationship:

"I want you... but just for the holidays"
When you just need someone to keep you warm during the winter nights, go for thoughtful but practical:

Holiday themed gifts: A Christmas ornament or a candle says, "I'm considerate and have good taste" but does not imply a commitment of any sort.

Food: Something edible makes people feel happy for now, and then they forget about it in a couple of weeks. That's similar to how you'd like the relationship to go.

Events: Try something intangible, like tickets to a concert or ice skating event. You will impress your new not-so-special someone long enough to keep the fire burning through the holidays. Oh, and don't spring for good seats, or you will have to get a Valentine's Day gift.

"I want you... forever"
This situation can be tricky and calls for very careful scrutiny of your relationship. You feel this way, but will your feelings be reciprocated? If you decide the other party's got it bad for you too, go all out:

Mix It Up: Give "lots of different things" such as clothes, a DVD, a CD, a book, some flowers.... It could get pricey, so be sure you are committed to this commitment. Plus, when you buy a bunch of little things, it does not make you look so bad when you screw up on some of them so be sure to include gift receipts also.

Take A Trip: Planning a trip together is a great way to say you're serious, especially if you plan it for later, like January. Plus, it's a gift you can both give each other so you don't have to worry that your gifts will be unbalanced. For example, you are unwrapping a new and expensive bracelet while she politely thanks you for the knitted stocking cap.

Jewelry: If you're up for it, nothing says, "I'm not just a jerk who wants your body" like jewelry. But since you just started dating, you may not know her taste just yet. If you're determined to make a grand statement, think earrings, a necklace or a bracelet; stay away from rings, which have tendencies to send an entirely different message.

Most important of all, don't let something as trivial as a gift ruin your holidays — or a potentially great relationship. Just apply the formula, and determine the message you want to send and have a great time dating during the holiday season.

Chapter: 68

"Voice Perception"

A great voice can be a huge turn-on. A man's deep voice or a woman's sexy voice can evoke one image, while a nasal whine can be an annoyance and will provoke a very different image. And it is very important that your voice is in check as well. This can be done simply by video taping yourself talking and reviewing the tape and practicing until you have corrected the problem.

Beyond that, here are a few insights that you can get from voice perception beyond those presented in written form? These are three tips that can help you understand the hidden messages in someone's voice:

Enthusiasm and Energy is Audible
Imagine for a minute your future could be riding on this person trying to pick you up or ask you out for a date. Certainly you would expect there to be some excitement and enthusiasm in their voice, right? If they are not excited about you, something is not right.

Watch out for anyone whose profile lists lots of sports and other high-energy activities but sounds like one of the living dead. Keep your ears open for someone that sounds upbeat, enthusiastic, and eager to make new connections.

Listen For Honesty - This is great advice!
The majority of people that you are going to meet both online and off are genuinely, good and honest people looking to meet other sincere people. Still, it's smart to listen for telltale hesitation on

certain key words (especially those related to marital status or commitment status).

Mispronunciation of the words that so impressed you in the text profile could also indicate that this person is not quite the intellectual that you had imagined they would be. A defensive tone or halting delivery is not a great sign, either. Trust your instincts and avoid anyone whose voice raises your suspicions or lowers your comfort level.

Charisma and Style Counts
On top of all the other factors that you need to take into consideration, communication chemistry has to be there, too. Do you like the tone, or speed at which the person you are talking to speaks? Is his/her accent or vocal quality appealing to you? Do you feel "comfort and warmth" in this voice? Does their laugh make you smile?

When you constantly find yourself thinking, wow, I really want to talk with this person again, you know you are on to something potentially great. So take everything you have learned and apply it and go for it!

Chapter: 69

"Online Dating Forums"

Some of the highest rated online dating forums to use for meeting people through the Internet as of Dec 18th 2009 include:

(In no certain order)

Match.com
Chemistry.com
PerfectMatch.com
Yahoo Personals
Eharmony.com
OkCupid.com
PlentyofFish.com
CasualKiss.com
Lavalife.com
DateHookUp.com
WooMe.com
ConnectingSingles.com
BookOfMatches.com
MatchDoctor.com

Chapter: 70

"How To Protect Yourself At All Times"

1. Use a service like http://orders.netdetective.net/cgi-bin/shop.cgi or www.SentryLink.com or http://datechecker.com/ or www.saferdates.com to do a criminal background check and/or credit check before meeting up with someone or deciding to get too involved. Better to be safe than sorry!

2. Trust your gut instinct at all times

3. Never take unnecessary risks

4. Never disclose all of your information (especially personal information)

5. Work the new relationship buildup in various stages (time and distance is your safety shield) you will learn more about relationship buildup by reading this book.

6. Avoid putting yourself in a vulnerable or compromising position that goes against your gut instincts

7. Always let someone else know where you are going, who you are going to be with, and what time to expect you back. Also leave their contact information if circumstances warrant.

8. Always call your contact when you arrive and when you leave (keep them informed).

9. Set a specific exit time and use it as a fall-back if needed (I have to be home by 10PM). If you decide to stay longer, well then that is OK too!

10. Ask for references of both sexes (male and female) if circumstances warrant.

11. Always meet in open and populated places where other people can see you for safety reasons.

12. Set a specific time-frame to meet to use as an exit strategy if needed

13. Bring a friend along with you if the circumstances warrant.

14. Never be afraid or embarrassed to cancel a date at the last moment if something does not feel right. This is your right and it has to be your CHOICE! Just tell them an emergency has come up and you have got to reschedule! Tell them you will call them once you are done! And Go! The NEXT step is up to you...so CHOOSE wisely!

Chapter: 71

"How To Verify Someone's Online Profile"

How to verify someone's online profile - Criminal background checks and credit reference checks should be conducted on anyone you are seriously considering getting involved with these days. You never know who you are going to meet and how nice they sound and how convincing they are. Well the truth of the matter is that if they sincerely care about you and your safety and happiness, they will not object to allowing you to conduct a criminal background check.

In fact they should be pretty understanding and happy that you have demonstrated yourself as intelligent enough to do the right thing. This should make them feel even more comfortable wanting to be with you unless they have something to hide from you. Either way you want to know for certain who you are about to get involved with.

You can use either of the following services to do background checks:
http://orders.netdetective.net/cgi-bin/shop.cgi
http://backgroundchecks.corragroup.com/
http://www.integrascan.com/?cj=1&AID=10753276&PID=3803363

So the next time you are ready to take the big leap forward in you new relationship, remember to protect yourself and run a background check and verify the person's identity, address, marital status, profession, and if necessary their credit.

Protect yourself at all times by CHOOSING to err on the side of caution!

Chapter: 72

"The Best Way To Transition From Chatting To Meeting In Person"

The best way to transition from chatting to meeting in person - is to first spend enough time chatting with and getting to know the person intimately enough to where you both feel comfortable wanting to meet each other in person.

Next, you want to spend some quality time on the phone talking to one another getting to know your likes and dislikes, hobbies, family history, marital status and situation. Then if you still feel comfortable about the prospect of meeting, set a casual date and see how things go. Remember to use the line for getting to know each other better. This is a great way to break the ice and begin transitioning from just chatting and talking on the phone to seeing each other in person. The key here is to be patient and not pushy. You need to build a level of trust that makes the other person feel comfortable stepping out of their comfort zone in order for them to take that leap of faith.

By moving the relationship forward in this patient and methodical way, you increase your chances of having a great time once you do get together and reduce your risk of possibly wasting your time and money. Both of which are expensive.

So the next time you are ready to transition from chatting to meeting in person, be patient, build up a certain level of trust, and make your first date fun and exciting so the other person will want to go on more dates with you. Do this gradually and always remember to think of how the other person feels since they do not know you that well yet. Make them feel as comfortable as possible.

Chapter: 73

"The Best Places To Meet"

The best places to meet for the first time in person are Coffee houses, donut shops, ice cream parlors, shopping mall food courts, nothing real fancy or expensive. Definitely want to meet in a well lit area with plenty of lighting preferably in public where other people can see you for safety reasons. Another idea is to ask the person to stand in a specific spot or location while waiting for you to arrive so you'll know exactly who they are before they know who you are. This gives you the upper hand on safety because you can see them from a distance and make body language assessments, facial assessments, and observation assessments. All of which helps your gut instinct make its final decision.

The objective is to first make sure you are still interested and on board with this person and want to continue moving forward with the relationship. Trust me, I've spent plenty of money and wasted enough of my time when all along my gut feeling was telling me to cut it short and leave. Of course being Mr. Nice Guy, I opt to stay and be polite and waste my time and money. Looking back, I should have listened to my gut feelings and left!

Chapter: 74

"Setting Guidelines For The First Time You Meet"

This is typically a very good idea for the very first time you step out to meet someone new. The best way to structure it is to let the other person know that you would like to meet up for coffee or tea for about 30 minutes to give each of you a little time to get to know each other better before getting too involved or serious with each other. If after the initial 30 minutes has passed and you feel comfortable with staying longer, feel free to convey your feelings and ask the other person to join you.

If on the other hand you do not feel comfortable for any reason, and do not want to stay longer, let your date know that you have enjoyed spending some time with them getting to know them more and that you need to get going for now and will speak with them later in the evening or tomorrow. Basically you want to let them down easily and be able to get away safely.

As a rule of thumb, you should always have your first date somewhere out in the public where other people can see you and help you if needed. This helps the other person remain calm and feel more comfortable and allows them to focus on being their self. Besides, this is what you are really after, this way you can see how they really are and then make your final decision about them.

They might be a hermit crab at home and completely opposite when they get out or vice versa. You need to get a good feel of who they are, how they act, and what their relationship goals are. You may find out that they are just drifting along in life aimlessly. If so, you need to reevaluate who you are with to what you want out of a relationship and none of this can take place until you have set guidelines to meet up with each other out in public to gain a better understanding of how compatible you will be and how this person really acts while out in public.

Chapter: 75

"The End Result"

The End Result – Ultimately, only you will know what end result you have in mind. Everyone else will have their opinions, perceptions, and ideas of what they think your end result is going to be or should be, but only you will know for certain. With that in mind, you have got to make a commitment to keep your focus on your end result no matter what anyone else might think or say about you. One of the biggest turn-offs I find in other people is their accepted belief to sell themselves short of what they are truly capable of accomplishing mostly because they have put more belief in what other people have told them what they cannot accomplish instead of truly believing in themselves and persistently focusing on what they can accomplish.

There are several philosophies that I have learned to live by that help me to stay focused on and keep my commitments no matter what anyone else says or thinks about me. And believe me, I have found out that people are very opinionated about my decisions, and actions, and that is ok with me, because ultimately I know what I am going after and what I want the end result to be and I have made a commitment to myself that nothing will distract my attention from achieving it. These important philosophies are:

1. "We become what we think about." Not only is this a philosophy, it is a proven fact. You may have heard the saying..."if you can control the space between your ears (your brain) then you can control destiny" This implies being in control of your mind and thoughts...

and everyone is in total control of their own thoughts whether they want to believe it or not. If someone does not believe that they are in total control of their own thoughts, then tell me who is? A better way to look at and understand this concept is to realize that we are the sum total of the embodiment of our thoughts up to this point in our life. Tomorrow, next week, next month, next year and so on, we will be the sum total of the embodiment of our thoughts at that point in time. We are where we are in our lives at this given moment because of what we have chosen to believe, think about and focus our attention on. This may be uncomfortable for some people to accept but it is a proven fact and once they realize and accept this fact, they can begin to change their lives for the better simply by changing their thoughts and what they focus on. "We become what we think about."

2. "We move in the direction of our most dominant thought." Think of your mind as a compass and whichever way the needle is pointing, is the direction that you are moving in. Here again, control and focus your thoughts and you will begin moving in that direction. Whether good or bad, our subconscious mind does not know the difference. It only knows that this is the direction that we must move in. Hence, if your dominant thought is on finding the perfect soul mate, you will begin moving in that direction and eventually find the person you have dreamed of. If your thoughts are very focused, you will find the ideal person quicker, if your thoughts are fragmented it will take longer. This process works the same for everyone and has no favorites. The quickest way to get what you want is to realize that you are in control of your thoughts and then begin to control and focus your thoughts, and then you will begin moving in that direction. "We move in the direction of our most dominant thought."

3. "The quality of my attention determines the quality of my time." I actually created this proven philosophy after years of experiencing varying degrees of quality of time. I realized that the more focus and attention (quality) I

put into whatever I was doing at any given time, the more I seemed to enjoy the time I spent in whatever I was doing. This happened because the more I focused on what I was doing the more I enjoyed doing it. If I give 100% of my attention to what I am doing, then I seem to enjoy the time more. This is especially true for engaging in conversations with other people. Mainly because of the subconscious law of psychological reciprocity. That is, people will give back to you in like kind what you give to them. Hence, give them 100% of your attention they will give you 100% of their attention in return. Give them 50% and they will give you 50% and so on. Pay them a sincere compliment and they will feel psychologically obligated to pay you a sincere compliment in return. If you want to improve the quality of your time, improve the quality of your attention. "The quality of my attention determines the quality of my time."

4. "Be choosy what you set your heart upon, for if you want it badly enough, you will get it." The problem that most people have is in not knowing how to get what they want. That can be taught through reading and understanding this and other books how to get whatever they desire. The problem is that most people do not know what they want and therefore run aimlessly through life until they discover something exciting that grabs their attention for a short period of time. When this gets old, they are off running aimlessly again. The key is in deciding on what you want to go after, controlling your thoughts, focusing your attention, and giving it 100% of your attention until you obtain it. Once you have what you are going after, decide on what you want to achieve next and go for it. By following this formula, you will achieve or get what you are going after every time. "Be choosy what you set your heart upon, for if you want it badly enough, you will get it."

These philosophies help me keep my focus on what I have set out to accomplish without worrying about someone else's opinion or thoughts. The reason I mention this is because I learned a long time ago that just like in a football game, in life, your opportunity is not over until the clock runs out and that other people will become very jealous of your enthusiasm and decisive attitude towards accomplishment. There have been so many occasions for me where I was about to give up on what I had set out to accomplish because it seemed nearly impossible for me to accomplish my goals or that time was running out. Ultimately though, I stuck to my philosophies and kept my focus and sometimes I pulled it off. Albeit, sometimes right at the very last moment. So never give up.

My belief in these philosophies has proved to me over and over again that sometimes in life you must absolutely beyond all doubts keep your commitments to your focus and never allow anyone or anything to deter you from what you want your end result to be. Whether it is to become rich, finish your degree, land the perfect job, start your own company, find the perfect date, get married, or have a family, you have got to be absolutely committed to the end result. There is no in-between and there are lots of people in this world that do not want to see you succeed or surpass them, so as a result, they will attempt to sabotage your psyche by telling you how difficult something may be, or you may be wasting your time, or some other negative comment, gesture, or laughter to deter you from accomplishing your end result. Whatever the case may be, keep your focus and always remember it is your life and therefore it is your CHOICE, you are in charge, and it is your happiness not theirs, that you are striving for.

I actually found out that the best way to approach a new end result that I wanted to accomplish is to keep it to yourself and then tell other people after you have accomplished it. This way nobody can steal your enthusiasm for your accomplishment. If you feel absolutely certain that there are people you can share your new goal with that will be positive and supportive, by all means share it with them. If they attempt to offer you suggestions or advice, listen to them and by all means stay committed to your end result. This does not mean that you should not be adaptable or flexible. Certainly, if along your path you discover a better or more reasonable way to reach your end result, you want to be open-minded enough to think outside of the box, and look at things with a fresh new perspective as opposed to a fixed preconceived belief on how things have to be.

After all, half of the fun in reaching the end result is in discovering new and different ways of doing things. Whatever the case, do not let someone else steal your opportunity. Just because something did not work for someone else does not mean that it will not work for you and vice versa. At first, almost everyone that found out that I met my wife Rose through the Internet thought I was nuts and felt that I was getting myself into more trouble than I could handle. Good thing I did not tell them until after I had already met her. I could only imagine what they would have said or thought of me if had told them before I met her. As it turns out, they absolutely love her and think the world of her. Best of all, I was able to use the Internet to find exactly the person I was looking to meet because I was committed to the end result! It all started with a little determination and a lot of persistence.

One of the other amazing things I have learned along the way in staying committed to accomplishing end results is that by remaining open-minded and learning to look at things with a fresh new perspective, your mind begins to grow exponentially in the belief and confidence of what it can achieve. After a while, you find yourself going through life without any limits placed on your abilities and soon after, other people notice your new enthusiasm and begin to have more respect for you because they envy what you have discovered about yourself.

Chapter: 76

"Final Word"

Above everything else, your safety and security are the most important factors that need to be taken into consideration at all times! You can always find another person, or go on another date as long as you are alive. So do not take any unnecessary chances or risks that you feel uncomfortable about. Besides, anyone that truly cares about you and has your best interest at heart, will not ask you to put yourself in any kind of harms way. Realize that you ALWAYS have a CHOICE and Learn to trust your instincts.

Good Luck to you and all of your relationship endeavors! Reflect back on the knowledge covered in this book to both protect yourself at all times and continue improving on your relationship skills. Congratulations to you for taking the right step towards improving all of your relationships. Your new and exciting journey is just beginning! Review these chapters from time to time to help remind you of these valuable lessons designed to help improve all of your relationships.

Likewise, if you know of someone struggling with their relationships, or just cannot seem to find the right person to marry or get involved with, gift them a copy of this book and help them get on the right track for having improved and more meaningful relationships. Who knows maybe one day they will return the favor for you. For contact information and any updates about this book, please visit our website at www.PsychologyOfCyberDating.com .

Thank you and may you have only the best in all of your relationships from now on!

ROBERT A. DAVENPORT grew up as the youngest of 12 kids on a small 5 acre farm in Hanover, Virginia raising chickens, ducks, goats, pigs, cows, and horses, while maintaining our own vegetable garden, and constantly cutting firewood to keep warm during the winter months. Needless to say growing for me up was extremely hard work until I left home at the age of 22.

I remember my life being filled with constant struggles and very little idle time. There was always something else that needed to be done, and whatever little time I had left over was spent working for neighboring farmers to make enough money to buy my own school clothes from the age of 12 onward.

Being the youngest of 12 kids I was always picked on, made fun of, and harassed by my older siblings. Little did they realize how much they were helping to shape me in to becoming a better person later in my life. To my siblings, their daily torture to me was just business as usual until they each got old enough to either run away from home or become brave enough to venture out on their own. To me it was my wake up call to figure out a better path in life and as a result I became determined to learn from all of their mistakes and make a better life for myself.

Physically I could not compete with my older siblings, so I had to learn to be quick with my thoughts in order to out think them and learn to use a lot of psychology to get through each day without getting beat up or made fun of as much as I got older. As a result, I became a master at reading body language, understanding what people were really saying by the way they used certain words and learned to identify and avoid danger whenever possible.

It is through these hard life lessons that I endured over the years that have allowed me to fine tune and hone my relationship skills that I share with you throughout this book. I pray that you take them very seriously and that you never have to go through the experiences I went through to learn them. Thank you and may God bless you with loving and lasting relationships.